Robotics in Plastic and Reconstructive Surgery

Jesse C. Selber

Editor

Robotics in Plastic and Reconstructive Surgery

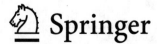 Springer

Editor
Jesse C. Selber
Department of Plastic Surgery
M.D. Anderson Cancer Center
Houston, TX
USA

ISBN 978-3-030-74246-1   ISBN 978-3-030-74244-7   (eBook)
https://doi.org/10.1007/978-3-030-74244-7

This Springer imprint is published by the registered company Springer Nature Switzerland AG
The registered company address is: Gewerbestrasse 11, 6330 Cham, Switzerland

This book is dedicated to the pioneering men and women of RAMSES (Robotic Assisted Microsurgery and Endoscopy Society), advancing the cause of robotic reconstruction since 2009.

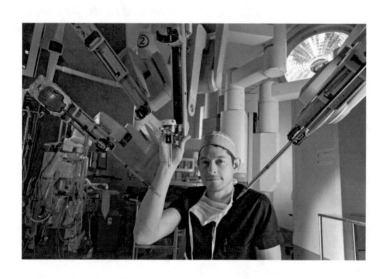

Preface

It has been my privilege to write and edit this book on robotic plastic and reconstructive surgery. We are in a time of great change. A global pandemic has required us to work differently, more remotely, and think in innovative ways about how we approach traditional problems. Surgical robotics removes the surgeon from much of the direct contact with the patient, and it is a fitting time to release a book which highlights these techniques as they apply to reconstructive surgery.

Originally, robotic surgical research was funded by NASA and the military to facilitate remote operations in forward areas and near-space, where surgical subspecialists are in short supply. It turned out that these remote applications were not immediately practical, and the technology was licensed to Intuitive Surgical, maker of the DaVinci, for minimally invasive surgery. The company designed their first-generation surgical robot for minimally invasive cardiac surgery. Although this application never gained a strong foothold, a group of innovative urologists applied the platform to prostate surgery, and the modern era of robotic surgery was born.

At this point in history, robotic surgery has come to dominate minimally invasive applications in many of the surgical subspecialties. Reconstructive efforts have been some of the last to be fully developed. This book is dedicated to those efforts. As you will see in the following pages, robotic reconstructive surgery has begun to gain momentum in several key areas which we will feature in this book. The chapters within contain applications in plastic surgery, but also in other types of reconstruction such as orthopedics and urology. Some of these are relevant because of either cross-over with plastic surgery practice, as in some of the orthopedic work, or analogous function, as in the luminal anastomoses in urology.

Minimally invasive surgery (MIS) is only one, albeit important benefit of a surgical robot. Several applications that highlight this function are contained within the book, such as the robotic rectus harvest and latissimus harvest. These have permitted the elimination of larger incisions from open surgery, analogous to the transition from the laparotomy to MIS. Similarly, we feature robotic surgery of the brachial plexus as an example of how treatment paradigms can change. In this case, the ability to not only explore but perform minimally invasive nerve repair and grafting may allow early exploration and repair to replace watchful waiting as the primary approach to closed brachial plexus injuries.

The other benefit of surgical robotics is precision. In reconstructive surgery, almost everything we do requires high levels of precision. The robot has 100%

tremor elimination, and up to 5:1 motion scaling, endowing it with super-human precision. Robotic microsurgery has emerged as the quintessential example of how this can be applied to enhance surgeon ability and benefit patients. In this book, we highlight both the learning curve of robotic microsurgical training and the advantages of micro-robotics in a busy, microsurgery practice. In addition, new technologies are emerging to meet this need more specifically. These new robotic microsurgical platforms promise to revolutionize microsurgical techniques and expand our ability to anastomose smaller and smaller structures such as lymphatics.

One of the more exciting and recent advances in this book are the robotic mastectomy and the robotic DIEP flap. The nipple sparing mastectomy (NSM) has beguiled breast surgeons for years because of the difficulty in accessing areas of the breast remote from the incision. With robotic NSM, this problem has promise of a solution. Breast reconstruction using the DIEP flap has been the enduring standard for autologous breast reconstruction for the last 20 years, but very little advancement has been made in the primary drawback to this operation: disruption of the abdominal wall. Using the roboDIEP, we are for the first time able to offer all the advantages of the DIEP and the length and caliber of its pedicle through an MIS approach with a very small fascial incision. This should change the game in abdominal wall morbidity resulting from the open DIEP.

Transoral robotic surgery is a unique area that has been developed by the head and neck surgeons to treat early stage cancer. Some of the more exciting but unexplored applications of TORS, however, are in cleft surgery and velopharyngeal dysfunction. In this book, we explore this technique and how it may change the way these surgeries are currently approached.

Robotic plastic surgery is still in its early developmental phase, but we will soon enter a steep part of the technology development curve that will provide us with smaller, more organic machines, augmented reality systems, surgical decision algorithms, much higher levels of precision, life-like haptics, and processing speeds beyond our imaginations. This is a very exciting time to be a robotic plastic surgeon. The chapters in this book represent some of the early forays into this new and exciting discipline. I invite the reader to allow their imagination to wander, not only to the present applications in robotic plastic surgery, but to the amazing possibilities that lay in the future.

Houston, TX, USA   Jesse C. Selber

Contents

Contributors

Yelena Akelina Microsurgery Research and Training Laboratory, Columbia University, New York, NY, USA

Taiba Alrasheed Department of Plastic Surgery, University of Texas, MD Anderson Cancer Center, Houston, TX, USA

Ghufran Alshaikh Maastricht University, Maastricht, The Netherlands

Chad M. Bailey Division of Proliance Surgeons, Plastic & Reconstructive Surgeons, Renton, WA, USA

Alberto Ballestín Microsurgery Department, Jesús Usón Minimally Invasive Surgery Centre, Cáceres, Spain

Tumor Microenvironment Laboratory, Institut Curie Research Center, Paris, Orsay, France

Sarah N. Bishop Department of Plastic Surgery, MD Anderson Cancer Center, Houston, TX, USA

Raimondo Cau Microsure, Eindhoven, The Netherlands

Mark W. Clemens Department of Plastic Surgery, MD Anderson Cancer Center, Houston, TX, USA

James M. Drake University of Toronto, The Hospital for Sick Children, Toronto, ON, Canada

Mohamed Etafy Avant Concierge Urology & University of Central Florida, Winter Garden, FL, USA

Alazhar Faculty of Medicine, Asyut, Egypt

David M. Fisher University of Toronto, The Hospital for Sick Children, Toronto, ON, Canada

Christopher R. Forrest University of Toronto, The Hospital for Sick Children, Toronto, ON, Canada

Ali Ghanem Group for Academic Plastic Surgery, The Blizard Institute, Queen Mary University of London, London, UK

Ahmet Gudeloglu Hacettepe University, Ankara, Turkey

Marco Innocenti Careggi University Hospital, Florence, Italy

Geraldine T. Klein Eisenhower Medical Association, Rancho Mirage, CA, USA

Thomas Lendvay University of Washington and Seattle Children's Hospital, Seattle, WA, USA

Philippe Liverneaux Department of Hand Surgery, SOS Main, CCOM, University Hospital of Strasbourg, FMTS, University of Strasbourg, Strasbourg, France

Thomas Looi University of Toronto, The Hospital for Sick Children, Toronto, ON, Canada

Richard A. Mendelson Keiser University Graduate School, Ft. Lauderdale, FL, USA

Tom J. M. van Mulken Maastricht University Hospital, Maastricht, The Netherlands

Sıjo J. Parekattıl Avant Concierge Urology & University of Central Florida, Winter Garden, FL, USA

John C. Pedersen Plastic Surgery, Cleveland Clinic, Akron, OH, USA

Louis L. Pisters The University of Texas MD Anderson Cancer Center, Houston, TX, USA

Dale J. Podolsky University of Toronto, The Hospital for Sick Children, Toronto, ON, Canada

Savitha Ramachandran KK Women's and Children's Hospital, Singapore, Singapore

Lars Johan M. Sandberg Oslo University Hospital, Rikshospitalet, Telemark Health Trust Skien, Norway, Oslo, Norway

Nicola Santelmo Department of Thoracic Surgery, University Hospital of Strasbourg, Strasbourg, France

Benjamin Sarfati Institut Gustave Roussy, Villejuif, France

Rutger M. Schols Maastricht University Hospital, Maastricht, The Netherlands

Jesse C. Selber Department of Plastic Surgery, MD Anderson Cancer Center, Houston, TX, USA

James Smartt Bucky Plastic Surgery, Philadelphia, PA, USA

Samuel Struk Institut Gustave Roussy, Villejuif, France

Hannah Teichmann VP Clinical Development and Medical Affairs, MMI SpA, Pisa, Italy

Joost A. G. N. Wolfs Maastricht University Hospital, Maastricht, The Netherlands

Karen W. Wong Riff University of Toronto, The Hospital for Sick Children, Toronto, ON, Canada

Fred Xavier Orthopedic Surgery, Biomedical Engineering, Cincinnati, OH, USA

Alice S. Yao Division of Plastic and Reconstructive Surgery, Department of Surgery, Icahn School of Medicine at Mount Sinai, New York, NY, USA

Part I
Training and Evaluation

Robotic Microsurgical Training

1

Savitha Ramachandran, Taiba Alrasheed, Alberto Ballestín⦿,
Yelena Akelina, and Ali Ghanem

The evolution of robotic platforms in the field of reconstructive surgery has enabled its applications in microvascular surgery, allowing two main advantages: enhanced visualization and improved precision [1, 2]. Robotic applications in microsurgery have been reported in the literature since the turn of the century, and robotic-assisted microvascular surgery in the last decade has been demonstrated to be feasible and advantageous particularly in intra-oral reconstructive surgery, where access is limited [3]. Robotic microsurgery has many theoretical advantages, complete tremor elimination and up to 5 to 1 motion scaling make the surgical robot capable of super-human levels of precision. In no area is this precision more important than in microsurgery [4, 5]. Several surgeons are already using the surgical robot to perform microsurgical techniques ranging from peripheral nerve anastomoses, vasectomy reversals, flap harvest, microvascular anastomoses, and lymphovenous bypass surgery [2, 5–8].

S. Ramachandran
KK Women's and Children's Hospital, Singapore, Singapore
e-mail: savitha.ramachandran@singhealth.com.sg

T. Alrasheed
Department of Plastic Surgery, University of Texas, MD Anderson Cancer Center, Houston, TX, USA

A. Ballestín (✉)
Microsurgery Department, Jesús Usón Minimally Invasive Surgery Centre, Cáceres, Spain

Tumor Microenvironment Laboratory, Institut Curie Research Center, Paris, Orsay, France
e-mail: balles_rodriguez@hotmail.com, alberto.ballestinrodriguez@curie.fr

Y. Akelina
Microsurgery Research and Training Laboratory, Columbia University, New York, NY, USA
e-mail: ya67@cumc.columbia.edu

A. Ghanem
Group for Academic Plastic Surgery, The Blizard Institute, Queen Mary University of London, London, UK

© Springer Nature Switzerland AG 2021
J. C. Selber (ed.), *Robotics in Plastic and Reconstructive Surgery*,
https://doi.org/10.1007/978-3-030-74244-7_1

As this technology rapidly advances, skill acquisition for the next generation of reconstructive microsurgeons must keep up at the same rate in order to effectively utilize this technology to improve patient outcomes [9, 10].

Microsurgery Teaching Methods

Microsurgery training across the world is heterogeneous. Courses vary in duration, but most of the centers identified offer a 35–45 hours (5 days) training schedule [11]. Some offer an *advanced* course in addition to a *basic* course. There is considerable variation in the trainee-to-trainer ratio, which may prove to have an effect on the trainee's learning through immediate feedback. In view of this, the International Microsurgery Simulation Society (IMSS) was established in 2011 by a group of dedicated microsurgery educators, with a vision of promoting in microsurgery training and education and to assist with standardization of training [12].

Microsurgery is a very difficult and demanding surgical skill that requires careful, professional instruction and a lot of practice. Ideally, microsurgery needs to be taught in a specially designed clinical simulation laboratory utilizing quality operating room surgical microscopes, instrumentation, and sutures, as well as both non-animated and animated models, such as different plastic materials, chicken thighs, and live rats [13–16]. The skills obtained from a microsurgery course significantly improve surgical skills and thus, meaningfully advance the quality of surgical patient care.

The first goal of a basic microsurgery course is to teach the students to become comfortable with working with the surgical microscope on its different powers of magnification as well as handling micro instruments and micro sutures. Learning the ergonomics, such as posture and hand positioning, is imperative to this goal and can be learned while working on non-animated models. Once this is learned, surgeons proceed to complete the procedures that are required, which involves anastomoses performed on the rat vessels, approximately of 1 mm in diameter. Each exercise starts with the careful dissection of the vessels. Magnification is used every step of the way to ensure the gentleness and careful handling of the fragile tissues. Different suturing techniques are taught to complete end-to-end and end-to-side anastomoses, interpositional vein grafts, and epineurial repairs of the sciatic nerve. Attendees have to complete both arterial and venous anastomoses, gradually moving from arteries to veins and then to grafts and nerves to increase the difficulty of handling more fragile vascular tissue and performing more complex procedures.

Research into teaching methods has reported that small student to teacher ratios, high fidelity models, and self-assessment during courses accelerate the rate of microsurgery skill acquisition [17].

Currently, there is only one center offering training courses specific to robotic microsurgery. The STAN institute in France runs courses in robotic microsurgery once a year for trained microsurgeons interested in enlarging their repertoire of skills. The details of the course can be found on their website [18].

Whether one can transfer previous microsurgery skills to robotic microsurgery is another consideration in training. *Karamanoukian* et al. conducted a study where they compared microsurgical vascular anastomosis of fully trained vascular surgeons and mid-level surgical residents on the robotic system [19]. They found no significant difference between the groups, and so previous microsurgical experience did not seem to affect the learning curves on the robot. *Ramdhian* et al. compared learning curves of robotic anastomosis and standard microsurgical anastomosis on a robot and microsurgical naïve surgeon. Although the learning curve for standard microsurgical anastomosis was faster than for robotic anastomosis, the difference was not statistically significant [20].

From the literature, it is clear that the establishment of a competency-based microsurgery curriculum will lead to the development of a structured curriculum for robotic microsurgery education. The tools developed for microsurgery assessment and training have already been adapted for application in robotic microsurgery training [9, 21]. Currently, the main drawback for the use of robotic technology in microsurgery is its cost. The high cost is also a major limiting factor in robotic microsurgery training, evidenced by the paucity of robotic microsurgery courses available. A standard 1-week course in microsurgery averages $2000 USD [22], while the 1-week course in robotic microsurgery at the STAN institute costs $6000 USD. Most training centers do not have the infrastructure within their simulation labs for robotic microsurgery training, and different laboratory setups are required for teaching (Fig. 1.1). Nevertheless, as the technology advances and robotic applications become more cost-effective, robotic microsurgery is identified as a field that has massive potential for expansion. As such, all efforts to develop robotic microsurgery education should persevere. Furthermore, as we approach the era of surgical revalidation, standardization in education and training would facilitate development as well as maintenance of skills [10, 11, 23].

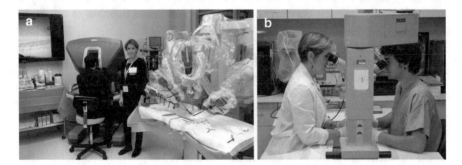

Fig. 1.1 Teaching of microsurgery and robotic microsurgery. (**a**) Laboratory training course setup using the da Vinci Surgical System (Intuitive Surgical, Sunnyvale, CA). (**b**) Laboratory training course setup for a microsurgery course

Assessment of Microsurgery and Robotic Microsurgery Skill Acquisition

Training and evaluation of skill acquisition in robotic microsurgery is firmly rooted in the literature available on traditional microsurgical training and education [9]. Microsurgical education used to be predominantly an apprenticeship (Halsteadian) model [24]. Lately, there has been widespread evidence to suggest that technical skills are best imparted systematically, with a standardized curriculum and measurable training endpoints [25–27]. As such, today the overwhelming trend in medical education, like other technically complex, high-stakes task training such as piloting a fighter jet or running a nuclear power plant, is leaning heavily toward competency-based training model. This shift toward competency-based surgical training, in the last decade, has inspired a plethora of publications supporting the development of a competency-based microsurgical curriculum [24, 28, 29]. Microsurgery educational research has focused on three main areas: (1) assessment of microsurgical skill acquisition, (2) simulation in training tools in microsurgery, and (3) teaching methods in microsurgery [11, 17, 30, 31].

Surgical skill assessment has two main functions: educational and evaluative. Assessment may aid learning as a formative assessment or assist evaluation as a summative assessment [25]. Miller's triangle best summarizes skill assessment in an individual. One of the earliest structured assessment tools for skill acquisition was developed by Kopta in 1971 [31]. This tool assigned a 3-point Likert scale to a checklist of steps for a particular task. *Reznick* et al. adapted this into a Structured Technical Skills Assessment Form (STSAF) and introduced it as a tool for surgical skill assessment [32]. He validated this and then further optimized it into the Objective Structured Assessment of Technical Skills (OSATS) [33].

Microsurgery demands fine motor skills and has a steep learning curve. In 2003, *Grober* et al. modified the OSATS and other previously validated checklists and adapted them for microsurgery assessment [33]. Since then, several authors have further modified and introduced global rating scales for objective assessment of microsurgical skill acquisition [34]. These objective assessment tools are crucial for the development of a competency-based curriculum. These tools have also been used to identify learning curves in microsurgery and hence function as a form of feedback to accelerate skill acquisition among residents [35].

For the assessment and training of robotic microsurgical skills, the same principles can be applied. The Structured Assessment of Robotic Microsurgery Skills (SARMS) evaluation system was introduced in 2014 [36]. The SARMS evaluation system is unique in that it combines previously validated skill assessment parameters for both microsurgery and robotic surgery [36]. The SARMS includes three parameters to assess conventional microsurgical skills, namely, (1) dexterity, (2) visuospatial ability, and (3) operative flow. The robotic skills incorporate five additional parameters, namely, (1) camera movement, (2) depth perception, (3) wrist articulation, (4) atraumatic tissue handling, and (5) atraumatic needle handling. Each parameter is scored from 1 to 5, with 1 being the worst and 5 the best. The

Table 1.1 Structured Assessment of Robotic Microsurgical Skills (SARMS)

Microsurgical skills

		1	2	3	4	5
Dexterity	Bimanual dexterity	Lack of use of non-dominant hand		Occasionally awkward use of non-dominant hand		Fluid movements with both hands working together
	Tissue handling	Frequently unnecessary force with tissue damage		Careful but occasional inadvertent tissue damage		Consistently appropriate with minimal tissue damage
Visuospatial ability	Micro suture placement	Frequently lost suture and uneven placement		Occasionally uneven suture placement		Consistently, delicately, and evenly spaced sutures
	Knot technique	Unsecure knots		Occasional awkward knot tying and improper tension		Consistently, delicately, and evenly placed sutures
Operative flow	Motion	Many unnecessary or repetitive moves		Efficient but some unnecessary moves		Economy of movement and maximum efficiency
	Speed	Excessive time at each step due to poor dexterity		Efficient time but some unnecessary or repetitive moves		Excellent speed and superior dexterity without awkward moves

Robotic skills

	1	2	3	4	5
1. Camera movement	Unable to maintain focus or suitable view		Occasionally out of focus and inappropriately view		Continually in focus and appropriate view
2. Depth perception	Frequent inability to judge object distance		Occasional empty grasp		Consistently able to judge spatial relations
3. Wrist articulation	Little or awkward wrist movement		Occasionally inappropriate wrist movement or angles		Continually using full range of endowrist motion
4. Atraumatic needle handling	Consistent bending/breakage of needle		Occasional bending/breakage of needle		Consistently undamaged needle
5. Atraumatic tissue handling	Consistent inappropriate grasping/crushing or over spreading of tissue		Occasional inappropriate grasping/crushing or over spreading of tissue		Consistently gentle handling of tissue

Reproduced with permission from Selber and Alrasheed [9]

overall performance and overall skill level are also independently assessed (Table 1.1).

To date, there is no consensus on a "gold standard" for the assessment of microsurgery, but the global rating scale remains the most easily accessible and applied [35]. Other objective assessment tools described and validated in the literature include hand motion analysis (HMA) [31, 37]. Hand motion analysis uses a tool that tracks hand motion through 3D space and has been pioneered and developed for laparoscopic surgery [37]. Currently, there are six published reports applying this technology to microsurgery training. The two technologies that have been developed for assessment of fine hand motor movements are hand motion electromagnetic (EM) sensors and video based with infra-red cameras that detect hand motion by measuring the distance to reflectors on the operator's hands [38, 39].

Virtual reality simulators have been developed and validated in laparoscopic surgery. Using outcome measures such as time to complete tasks and economy of movement, they have been able to demonstrate construct validity in laparoscopic surgery [40]. However due to lack of haptic feedback, its use has been limited in microsurgery assessment and training. The use of virtual reality simulator systems in robotic surgical training is well established in the surgical curriculum. There are six virtual reality simulators available for robot-assisted surgery: the daVinci Skills Simulator (dVSS), the Mimic dV Trainer (MdVT), the ProMIS simulator, the Simsurgery Educational Platform (SEP) simulator, the Robotic Surgical Simulator (RoSS), and the RobotiX Mentor (RM) [41, 42]. None of these platforms have explored robotic microsurgery simulation for skill acquisition, and this could be a potential tool used in the future of robotic microsurgery training and assessment [35].

Simulation Models

Simulation models for training is another area of research interest for microsurgery training. Once an ideal training model is established, a multitude of educational tasks can be accomplished, validating objective assessment tools, plotting of a learning curve as well as designing customized training models, and comparing curricula, trainees, and instructors.

Ilie et al. have classified microsurgery training models into five main groups [43]:

1. Basic manipulation, movement, and orientation in operative field
2. Knot placement/tying principles – apposition of edges, non-dominant hand usage, deformable volumes
3. Three-dimensional models
4. The real tissue experience
5. Virtual reality trainers

Synthetic low fidelity bench models, such as silicone tubes, are cost-effective and assist in the development of rudimentary skills such as scope or robot adjustment and instrument handling, but little has been reported about its predictive validity beyond these basic skills [44]. Some specific training platforms for robotic microsurgery learning in a laboratory have been developed (Fig. 1.2). Interestingly, the use of Lego as a bench tool has also been reported by *Parekattil* et al. [20]. More sophisticated simulation models such as a life-size intra-oral cavity have been

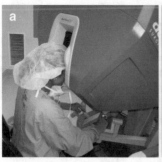
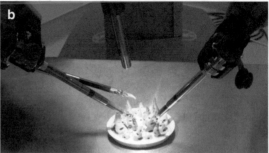

Fig. 1.2 Robotic microsurgery training laboratory. (**a**) Surgeon using da Vinci Surgical System console. (**b**) da Vinci Surgical System dry laboratory training platform

developed for simulation training in cleft surgery and can be explored for intra-oral robotic surgery [25].

A further step in simulation training is the integration of skills into a real-life surgical experience with convincing face validity [25]. Both anatomical and physiological components of the procedure must be simulated. Non-living animal models such as rat aorta and the chicken thigh or human cadavers are able to simulate the anatomical aspects of the procedure as to develop further skills in tissue handling and tissue dissection, but the physiological aspects of the procedure are not experienced using this model [14, 45]. For the full real-life experience, high fidelity models such as the live rat are critical in microsurgery training. Restrictions due to ethical concerns make these models increasingly more difficult to have access to, nonetheless, they are crucial to microsurgery training and skill acquisition. There are three main established surgical approaches for the microdissection of vessels and nerves and its suturing for the rat model: the neck, the abdomen, and the groin. With these three approaches, a surgeon can learn how to dissect and prepare micro-vessels from 0.5 to 2 mm working on different vessels: carotid arteries, jugular veins, aorta, cava vein, femoral vessels, and epigastric vessels. The trainees use these vessels to learn and practice conventional microsurgical techniques such as end-to-end, end-to-side anastomosis, interpositional vein graft, bypass, AV fistulas, and microvascular free flaps. In addition to vessels, the hindlimb of the rat is used to work on the sciatic nerve, where epineural or perineural neuroanastomosis techniques can be practiced. *Parakettil* et al. recommend use of the earthworms, while subsequently progressing to live animal models in the training of robotic microsurgery [20, 46].

Learning Curves in Microsurgery

With the establishment of objective assessment tools in microsurgery such as the global rating scales, learning curves in microsurgery were identified to demonstrate skill acquisition in the simulation lab, validate microsurgical simulation models, and to establish safe clinical thresholds for microsurgery [12, 47]. Learning curves are increasingly used in surgical training and education to denote the process of gaining knowledge and improving skills in performing a surgical procedure [21]. These tools provide an objective assessment of technical ability and a benchmark to compare surgical approaches and technologies. The learning curve is defined by the number of cases required to achieve technical competence at performing a particular surgery [30]. Although this end point is easy to measure, it is fundamentally low resolution in that it does not provide objective definitions of learning and is not a direct indicator of learning [48].

Attempting to define learning curves in a clinical setting is challenging [30]. Variation in patient anatomy, operative conditions, surgeon factors, and many other varying clinical situations introduce bias into the evaluation of the learner [47]. The microsurgical anastomosis is an ideal model for evaluating skills and defining a learning curve because it is a finite task with a straightforward sequence of steps [21, 34]. The use of synthetic vessels of a predetermined size and the performance of a specific technical method make the teaching model extremely reproducible, with minimal variations depending on the skill and alacrity of the learner.

By using this established model, *Alrasheed* et al. were able to demonstrate improvement in robotic microsurgical skill across a heterogeneous group of learners using SARMS [36]. All skill areas and overall performance improved significantly for each participant over several robotic microsurgery sessions. Operative time decreased over the study for all participants. The results showed an initial steep technical skill acquisition followed by more gradual improvement, and a steady decrease in operative times that ranged between 1.2 hours and 9 minutes. They found that prior experience with conventional microsurgery did in certain areas improve the acquisition of technical proficiency using the robotic system. All groups demonstrated an ability to gain proficiency in robotic microsurgical anastomosis with minimal robot-specific training, indicating that the technical aspects of robotic microsurgery can be gained by learners with no prior microsurgery experience. Because of the inherent benefit of the robotic surgical platform for microsurgery, there is considerable interest in defining its role. In order to do this in an organized, controlled, and systematic fashion, *Alrasheed* et al. developed a well-defined anastomotic model, a validated assessment tool, and a general sense of the trajectory of learning [36, 45].

The performance of robotic-assisted microsurgery show steep, but relatively short learning curves. The further development of robotic platforms and the improvement and adaptation of the microsurgery training curriculum will change the clinical indications of conventional and robotic microsurgery. These innovations will facilitate the learning of surgeons in increasingly advanced techniques and thus improve the treatment of patients.

References

1. Selber JC, Robb G, Serletti JM, Weinstein G, Weber R, Holsinger FC. Transoral robotic free flap reconstruction of oropharyngeal defects: a preclinical investigation. Plast Reconstr Surg. 2010;125(3):896–900.
2. Dobbs TD, Cundy O, Samarendra H, Khan K, Whitaker IS. A systematic review of the role of robotics in plastic and reconstructive surgery-from inception to the future. Front Surg. 2017;4:66.

3. Selber JC, Sarhane KA, Ibrahim AE, Holsinger FC. Transoral robotic reconstructive surgery. Semin Plast Surg. 2014;28(1):35–8.
4. Moorthy K, Munz Y, Dosis A, Hernandez J, Martin S, Bello F, et al. Dexterity enhancement with robotic surgery. Surg Endosc. 2004;18(5):790–5.
5. Parekattil SJ, Brahmbhatt JV. Robotic approaches for male infertility and chronic orchialgia microsurgery. Curr Opin Urol. 2011;21(6):493–9.
6. van Mulken TJM, Boymans C, Schols RM, Cau R, Schoenmakers FBF, Hoekstra LT, et al. Preclinical experience using a new robotic system created for microsurgery. Plast Reconstr Surg. 2018;142(5):1377–8.
7. Clemens MW, Kronowitz S, Selber JC. Robotic-assisted latissimus dorsi harvest in delayed-immediate breast reconstruction. Semin Plast Surg. 2014;28(1):20–5.
8. Facca S, Hendriks S, Mantovani G, Selber JC, Liverneaux P. Robot-assisted surgery of the shoulder girdle and brachial plexus. Semin Plast Surg. 2014;28(1):39–44.
9. Selber JC, Alrasheed T. Robotic microsurgical training and evaluation. Semin Plast Surg. 2014;28(1):5–10. https://doi.org/10.1055/s-0034-1368161.
10. Dulan G, Rege RV, Hogg DC, Gilberg-Fisher KM, Arain NA, Tesfay ST, et al. Developing a comprehensive, proficiency-based training program for robotic surgery. Surgery. 2012;152(3):477–88.
11. Leung CC, Ghanem AM, Tos P, Ionac M, Froschauer S, Myers SR. Towards a global understanding and standardisation of education and training in microsurgery. Arch Plast Surg. 2013;40(4):304–11.
12. Ghanem A, Kearns M, Ballestin A, Froschauer S, Akelina Y, Shurey S, et al. International Microsurgery Simulation Society (IMSS) consensus statement on the minimum standards for a basic microsurgery course, requirements for a microsurgical anastomosis global rating scale and minimum thresholds for training. Injury. 2020;51(Suppl 4):S126–30.
13. Shurey S, Akelina Y, Legagneux J, Malzone G, Jiga L, Ghanem AM. The rat model in microsurgery education: classical exercises and new horizons. Arch Plast Surg. [Review]. 2014;41(3):201–8.
14. Pafitanis G, Serrar Y, Raveendran M, Ghanem A, Myers S. The chicken thigh adductor profundus free muscle flap: a novel validated non-living microsurgery simulation training model. Arch Plast Surg. 2017;44(4):293–300.
15. Ballestin A, Casado JG, Abellan E, Vela FJ, Campos JL, Martinez-Chacon G, et al. A preclinical Rat Model for the study of ischemia-reperfusion injury in reconstructive microsurgery. J Vis Exp. [Video-Audio Media]. 2019;(153) https://doi.org/10.3791/60292.
16. Uson J, Calles MC. Design of a new suture practice card for microsurgical training. Microsurgery. [Evaluation Studies]. 2002;22(8):324–8.
17. Ghanem AM, Hachach-Haram N, Leung CC, Myers SR. A systematic review of evidence for education and training interventions in microsurgery. Arch Plast Surg. 2013;40(4):312–9.
18. Liverneaux PA, Hendriks S, Selber JC, Parekattil SJ. Robotically assisted microsurgery: development of basic skills course. Arch Plast Surg. 2013;40(4):320–6.
19. Karamanoukian RL, Bui T, McConnell MP, Evans GR, Karamanoukian HL. Transfer of training in robotic-assisted microvascular surgery. Ann Plast Surg. 2006;57(6):662–5.
20. Gudeloglu A, Brahmbhatt JV, Parekattil SJ. Robotic-assisted microsurgery for an elective microsurgical practice. Semin Plast Surg. 2014;28(1):11–9.
21. Lee JY, Mattar T, Parisi TJ, Carlsen BT, Bishop AT, Shin AY. Learning curve of robotic-assisted microvascular anastomosis in the rat. J Reconstr Microsurg. 2012;28(7):451–6.
22. Singh M, Ziolkowski N, Ramachandran S, Myers SR, Ghanem AM. Development of a five-day basic microsurgery simulation training course: a cost analysis. Arch Plast Surg. 2014;41(3):213–7.
23. Kearns MC, Baker J, Myers S, Ghanem A. Towards standardization of training and practice of reconstructive microsurgery: an evidence-based recommendation for anastomosis thrombosis prophylaxis. Eur J Plast Surg. 2018;41(4):379–86.
24. Balasundaram I, Aggarwal R, Darzi LA. Development of a training curriculum for microsurgery. Br J Oral Maxillofac Surg. 2010;48(8):598–606.

25. Atkins JL, Kalu PU, Lannon DA, Green CJ, Butler PE. Training in microsurgical skills: does course-based learning deliver? Microsurgery. [Evaluation Studies]. 2005;25(6):481–5.
26. Schaverien MV, Butler CE, Suami H, Garvey PB, Liu J, Selber JC. Interview scores correlate with fellow microsurgical skill and performance. J Reconstr Microsurg. 2018;34(3):211–7.
27. Ramachandran S, Ong YS, Chin AY, Song IC, Ogden B, Tan BK. Stepwise training for reconstructive microsurgery: the journey to becoming a confident microsurgeon in Singapore. Arch Plast Surg. 2014;41(3):209–12.
28. Ko JW, Lorzano A, Mirarchi AJ. Effectiveness of a microvascular surgery training curriculum for orthopaedic surgery residents. J Bone Joint Surg Am. 2015;97(11):950–5.
29. Komatsu S, Yamada K, Yamashita S, Sugiyama N, Tokuyama E, Matsumoto K, et al. Evaluation of the microvascular research center training program for assessing microsurgical skills in trainee surgeons. Arch Plast Surg. 2013;40(3):214–9.
30. Lascar I, Totir D, Cinca A, Cortan S, Stefanescu A, Bratianu R, et al. Training program and learning curve in experimental microsurgery during the residency in plastic surgery. Microsurgery. 2007;27(4):263–7.
31. Pafitanis G, Narushima M, Yamamoto T, Raveendran M, Veljanoski D, Ghanem AM, et al. Evolution of an evidence-based supermicrosurgery simulation training curriculum: a systematic review. J Plast Reconstr Aesthet Surg. 2018;71(7):976–88.
32. Grober ED, Hamstra SJ, Wanzel KR, Reznick RK, Matsumoto ED, Sidhu RS, et al. Laboratory based training in urological microsurgery with bench model simulators: a randomized controlled trial evaluating the durability of technical skill. J Urol. 2004;172(1):378–81.
33. Grober ED, Hamstra SJ, Wanzel KR, Reznick RK, Matsumoto ED, Sidhu RS, et al. The educational impact of bench model fidelity on the acquisition of technical skill: the use of clinically relevant outcome measures. Ann Surg. 2004;240(2):374–81.
34. Chan W, Niranjan N, Ramakrishnan V. Structured assessment of microsurgery skills in the clinical setting. J Plast Reconstr Aesthet Surg. 2010;63(8):1329–34.
35. Ramachandran S, Ghanem AM, Myers SR. Assessment of microsurgery competency-where are we now? Microsurgery. 2013;33(5):406–15.
36. Alrasheed T, Liu J, Hanasono MM, Butler CE, Selber JC. Robotic microsurgery: validating an assessment tool and plotting the learning curve. Plast Reconstr Surg. 2014;134(4):794–803.
37. Grober ED, Hamstra SJ, Wanzel KR, Reznick RK, Matsumoto ED, Sidhu RS, et al. Validation of novel and objective measures of microsurgical skill: hand-motion analysis and stereoscopic visual acuity. Microsurgery. [Research Support, Non-U.S. Gov't]. 2003;23(4):317–22.
38. Satterwhite T, Son J, Carey J, Echo A, Spurling T, Paro J, et al. The Stanford Microsurgery and Resident Training (SMaRT) scale: validation of an on-line global rating scale for technical assessment. Ann Plast Surg. 2014;72(Suppl 1):S84–8.
39. McGoldrick RB, Davis CR, Paro J, Hui K, Nguyen D, Lee GK. Motion analysis for microsurgical training: objective measures of dexterity, economy of movement, and ability. Plast Reconstr Surg. 2015;136(2):231e–40e.
40. Nayar SK, Musto L, Fernandes R, Bharathan R. Validation of a virtual reality laparoscopic appendicectomy simulator: a novel process using cognitive task analysis. Ir J Med Sci. 2019;188:963–71.
41. Whitehurst SV, Lockrow EG, Lendvay TS, Propst AM, Dunlow SG, Rosemeyer CJ, et al. Comparison of two simulation systems to support robotic-assisted surgical training: a pilot study (Swine model). J Minim Invasive Gynecol. 2015;22(3):483–8.
42. MacCraith E, Forde JC, Davis NF. Robotic simulation training for urological trainees: a comprehensive review on cost, merits and challenges. J Robot Surg. 2019;13(3):371–7.
43. Ilie VG, Ilie VI, Dobreanu C, Ghetu N, Luchian S, Pieptu D. Training of microsurgical skills on nonliving models. Microsurgery. [Research Support, Non-U.S. Gov't]. 2008;28(7):571–7.
44. Chan WY, Matteucci P, Southern SJ. Validation of microsurgical models in microsurgery training and competence: a review. Microsurgery. [Review]. 2007;27(5):494–9.
45. Shurey S, Akelina Y, Legagneux J, Malzone G, Jiga L, Ghanem AM. The rat model in microsurgery education: classical exercises and new horizons. Arch Plast Surg. 2014;41(3):201–8.

46. Brahmbhatt JV, Gudeloglu A, Liverneaux P, Parekattil SJ. Robotic microsurgery optimization. Arch Plast Surg. 2014;41(3):225–30.
47. Selber JC, Chang EI, Liu J, Suami H, Adelman DM, Garvey P, et al. Tracking the learning curve in microsurgical skill acquisition. Plast Reconstr Surg. 2012;130(4):550e–7e.
48. Darzi A, Smith S, Taffinder N. Assessing operative skill. Needs to become more objective. BMJ. 1999;318(7188):887–8.

Robotic Skills Assessment: Crowd-Sourced Evaluation in Surgery and Future Directions in Plastic Surgery

Thomas Lendvay and James Smartt

Introduction

A surgeon's technique directly drives patient outcomes [1]. Upwards of 400,000 people die each year from medical errors, a third of which are attributable to surgical errors. Thus, medical errors are the third leading cause of death in the United States, above diabetes, stroke, and trauma [2]. Recognizing that the Halsteadian model of training, whereby one or a few mentors decide the advancement track of a trainee, can create gaps in proficiency, educators have shifted to a more standardized and consensus-driven format for trainee advancement. Furthermore, hospitals trying to standardize credentialing processes are turning to more objective peer review technologies and services. The intention is to modulate and optimize all facets of clinical skill prior to clinicians making errors. In surgery, a clinical field heavily reliant on the technical skills of the provider, improvement efforts have targeted these skills in addition to cognitive skills improvement. The challenge in a country where 51,000,000 surgeries are performed annually is how are we going to scale the process of surgical skills assessment and feedback [3]. In this chapter, we highlight the evolution and validation of a rapid, scalable, practical technique appraisal technology – Crowd-Sourced Assessment of Technical Skills (CSATS).

T. Lendvay
University of Washington and Seattle Children's Hospital, Seattle, WA, USA
e-mail: Thomas.lendvay@seattlechildrens.org

J. Smartt (✉)
Bucky Plastic Surgery, Philadelphia, PA, USA
e-mail: smartt@drbucky.com

© Springer Nature Switzerland AG 2021
J. C. Selber (ed.), *Robotics in Plastic and Reconstructive Surgery*,
https://doi.org/10.1007/978-3-030-74244-7_2

The Current State of Assessment in Surgical Education

In the United States, there are roughly 135,000 practicing surgeons and another 20,000 surgical trainees [4, 5]. The Accredited Council of Graduate Medical Education (ACGME), which oversees and monitors the compliance of all residency programs, has provided a template for how trainees should be assessed throughout their training. The Milestones Project established in 2012 by Tom Nasca, CEO of the ACGME, employs core competency domains to determine the aptitude of a trainee. Surgical skill is a piece of one of the six core competencies, and the ACGME has left it to individual surgical disciplines and programs to create how they want to assess the technical skills sub-domains. Although each surgical discipline is governed by residency review committees (RRCs) which have distributed key milestones that all trainees in each discipline must meet, programs rely on individual faculty to "score" these milestones. This introduces inherent biases into the review process. The ACGME posts annual results of the ascending pattern of scores as trainees move through their training program, and it is expected that trainees advance such that their scores reach graduation level or above in most of their domains. Residency programs feel compelled to graduate trainees within their allotted residency timeframe, and it is difficult to remediate trainees beyond the prescribed graduation time for each program as additional resources, creative scheduling, and impacts on subsequently ascending trainees have to be reconciled.

Credentialing

Whereas in residency training, there is a framework for how trainees are to be assessed, in the practitioner environment, hospitals are completely on their own in credentialing surgeons. There are no standard credentialing guidelines in the United States. The current workflow for a hospital to credential and grant privileges to a surgeon for particular types of surgeries relies on residency graduation and peer recommendation letters (usually chosen by the entrant surgeon). More progressive and proactive hospitals employ proctoring systems where senior surgeons either within the same practice or hospital or external proctors come and shadow the new surgeon for a few cases to assess the surgeon's safety, judgment, and skill. Because experience of the surgeons has been associated with patient outcomes [6, 7], hospitals' credentialing bodies turn to case currency – how many particular cases a surgeon does annually – as a means to allow a surgeon to continue to perform certain procedures. Case currency cut-points are set arbitrarily and not based on evidence that these numbers translate to proficiency. Each surgeon attains skill at different paces and a one-size-fits-all methodology can be sub-optimal. When hospitals are determining a surgeon's aptitude when adopting new technologies, some hospitals require dry-lab and/or animate lab experiences in the new technology before signing off on the surgeon. Again, this is not based on evidence as much as on the sentiment that the surgeon has at least practiced *some* with this new device or technology or surgical approach before performing human surgery.

In addition to these efforts not being grounded in evidence, they are expensive and time-intensive. Hospitals which require proctoring must pay for the proctors that can run in the thousands of dollars [8, 9]. If the hospital chooses to use internal proctors, these proctoring clinicians must be removed from their revenue-generating practices for a period of time to do the proctoring. The internal proctors might also introduce more rating bias. For example, if the proctor is a senior partner in the same practice as the proctee, the incentive is to rapidly advance the junior partner so that he/she can start generating revenue. If the proctor is from a competing practice in the community, alternative or negative biases could be introduced. The proctor may be disincentivized to advance the proctee. Moreover, usually only one proctor is used in the evaluation process which can limit the generalizability of this proctor's assessments.

Outside of the United States, some countries employ a more rigorous process to certifying a surgeon's technical skill when embracing new technologies. In Japan, when a surgeon wishes to become credentialed for robotic-assisted surgeries, each surgeon must submit raw un-edited video to a central national agency made up of 42 surgical skills referees. These videos are watched by two independent referees blinded to the identity of the surgeon [10, 11]. The pass rate for this review process is 67% and after 8 years of the agency review, over 7000 hours of video had been assessed. This is extremely time-intensive and requires agreement of the two referees which does not always happen. Though the citizens of Japan can take some comfort that their 6000 plus minimally invasive surgeons within the country have been vetted through a unique and rigorous process, there are issues of scalability, cost, and politics were such a process to be rolled out in the United States. If such a process were to be tested, consensus on the optimal assessment tools would need to be reconciled.

Objective Structured Assessment

In 1996, Martin et al. established the Objective Structured Assessment of Technical Skills (OSATS) as a means to quantify the technical skills of trainees in an open dry-lab surgical setting [12]. This validated tool became the backbone of many subsequent surgical approach and surgical procedure assessment tools which are used today to add objectivity to the trainee and practitioner appraisal process. In the original OSATS study, the Toronto group deconstructed the technical skill of a surgeon into domains – bimanual dexterity, depth perception, tissue handling, efficiency, and autonomy. These domains can be graded by reviewers/educators/proctors using a Likert scale and have been shown to be reliable and valid when trying to discriminate levels of skill. Furthermore, many studies have confirmed that these core domains translate into surgical outcomes, both peri- and postoperatively [13, 14]. These domains can be applied to a number of surgical approaches – open, laparoscopic, microsurgical, endoscopic, and robotic-assisted [15, 16]. The OSATS system can also be applied across surgical subfields, including the majority of plastic and reconstructive surgery.

Barriers to OSATS

These tools are used for research studies when testing new surgical training interventions or technologies, and are employed when educators are trying to stratify levels of expertise [17, 18]. Although ideally suited for assessing proficiency, these tools are less commonly used in training programs for advancement or by hospital credentialing bodies for privileging for a number of reasons. To start, the original OSATS studies involved individual mentors directly observing the trainees in a live setting. This requires time from experts/proctors which removes them from their own clinical practices. And since the process cannot be blinded if the reviewer is watching the subject live, bias can be introduced making this less of an "objective" process and more subjective. A single review may not agree with another reviewers' appraisal were the organization be able to get many reviews performed for the same performance. Also, the reviewers themselves need to understand the rating tool/process, they need to be educated in the art of delivering feedback, and they need to be accepted as content experts – a designation that does not have any established benchmarks. When these barriers are combined, the result is the infrequent use of such assessment tools.

There are methods to mitigate many of these biases. For one, capturing video of a performance or surgery and having the video reviewed after the performance allows for blinding of the subject, may allow for an increased pool of reviewers, and may reduce the performance anxiety of the performer knowing that there is not someone looking over their shoulder and rating them. This is more difficult in open surgery where physical attributes of the performer are hard to blind and obtaining standard high-quality video can be challenging. In minimally invasive and endoscopic surgery, however, the ability to capture and save performance video has led to an expansion of objective assessment. The camera's eye of a robotic-assisted, laparoscopic, or endoscopic surgical approach inherently blinds a reviewer to the identity of performer.

In robotic-assisted surgery, Goh et al. validated a skills appraisal tool – Global Evaluative Assessment of Robotic Skills (GEARS) – which has been repeatedly tested in dry lab, animate lab, and human surgery environments. In fact, scores using the GEARS tool directly correlate with patient outcomes [14, 19]. The ubiquity of an assessment process, however, is determined by its practicality. And although the GEARS tool has enjoyed extensive validation, it still requires that (a) there is/are enough available raters, (b) the raters agree with each other, and (c) the raters provide timely feedback within the window when the feedback resonates with the evaluatee.

Crowd-Sourced Assessment of Technical Skills (CSATS)

In 2013, Birkmeyer et al. demonstrated that a skills assessment of a single performance of a surgeon could predict the surgeon's patient outcomes among an entire year's worth of patients from that surgeon [1]. Their group recruited 20 practitioners among a collaborative of bariatric surgeons who were interested in testing the hypothesis that peers could review and that their reviews could portend how well those surgeons' laparoscopic gastric bypass patients fared over the course of the year. Ten expert surgeons within the Michigan Bariatric Surgery Collaborative (MBSC) watched the individual surgeons' videos and rated them on technical skills based on a modified OSATS tool for laparoscopy. These data were adjusted for hospital, comorbidities of the patients, and other non-technical factors which could normally impact patient outcomes as well. They observed that surgeons who were rated in the bottom quartile of skill when compared to the top quartile had threefold higher complication rates, fivefold higher death rates, 30% longer operative times, and statistically significantly higher 30-day readmission rates. Not just in the patients whose videos were reviewed, but among the entire year of patients each clinician cared for. These findings finally provided empiric evidence that the technique of a surgeon drives patient outcomes. This laid the foundation for subsequent initiatives to help surgeons improve their skill through some type of surgical review process. The barrier that was not addressed or reconciled in the Birkmeyer et al. study was the review time. It took almost 1 year for all reviews to be completed for just 20 surgical cases. Such a feedback process if it were to be operationalized would need feedback on the order of days to weeks, not months to be effective to improve a surgeon's performance before their next cases. A system to rapidly and reliably rate performances is required.

Dry-Lab Validation

To test an alternative surgical skills assessment process, Chen et al. in 2014 described the use of non-surgeon assessors [20]. In their initial study, they amassed over 500 lay crowdworkers through the Amazon.com's Mechanical Turk crowdsourcing platform to review a single 2-minute video of a robotic-assisted laparoscopic intracorporeal dry-lab suturing task. The video had been extracted from a set of videos stratifying various performance levels from residents and robotic surgery faculty. The video had been rated as an above-average performance based of kinematic or surgical tool movement signatures which correlated with expertise. The video was distributed to the 501 crowdworkers and a panel of 10 expert robotic surgery faculty in a single institution. In order to hone the assessment skills of the reviewers, the authors eliminated reviewers who incorrectly answered a series of discrimination and attention questions as part of the initial survey. Those reviewers' data were not included in the analysis. The online survey that was posted to the reviewers included an attention question asking the reviewers to not answer the following question which asked them how attentive they were. If answered, their data were excluded from analysis as it suggested they were not paying attention. The following question showed a side-by-side video of two surgeons (one novice and one expert) performing a robotic-assisted objective transfer task. The reviewers were asked to choose which performer was better. If the reviewer answered the question incorrectly, their data were excluded from analysis. Finally, each reviewer was exposed to the short suturing video clip and was asked to score the performer using three domains from the GEARS tool – bimanual dexterity, depth perception, and efficiency, tissue handling – just as the expert surgeons rating the performance. Neither the expert surgeon raters, nor the Turkers (presumably mostly non-medically trained) were given any education about how to use of what the assessment tool was. They merely had to read the three domains, read the various anchor details for each number on the Likert scale and score the performance. After eliminating the reviewers from the analysis, scores were correlated between the average of the expert raters and the average of the Amazon Turkers. Nine out of ten expert raters were included as one expert got the objective transfer discrimination choice wrong and 409 Turkers' scores were included. The mean scores provided by the two rater cohorts out of a possible 15/15 were 12.21 for the experts and 12.11 for the crowdworkers, respectively. Furthermore, the shear volume of crowdworkers yielded a confidence interval within that of the expert reviewers. There also appeared to be disagreement among the expert raters. Some felt the performance was at the top of the scoring tool, while others felt that the performance was just above average. Each crowdworker was remunerated with $1.00 USD for doing the survey, whereas the faculty expert reviewers received no such compensation. The 501 crowdworkers completed the survey in less than 24 hours. It took the experts over 3 weeks to complete the brief survey. Because the authors were using crowdsourcing and using the OSATS principle, they called the survey process Crowd-Sourced Assessment of Technical Skills (CSATS).

These findings led to a subsequent validation study where White et al. demonstrated that crowdworkers could discriminate levels of skills [21]. In their study, videos from 49 surgeons ranging from novice residents to expert robotic surgery faculty were distributed in the same type of survey, this time to 3 expert reviewers and on average 30 crowdworkers for each 2-minute suturing video clip. Again, the survey included three of the technical skills domains from the GEARS tool with a possible score as high as 15/15 meaning the top skill demonstrated. Over 1500 crowdworker reviews were completed in under 9 hours, whereas it took the three expert surgeons over 3 weeks to complete their surveys. The average scores of the expert raters correlated extremely well with the average crowdworker scores ($R = 0.92$).

Another study by Holst et al. tested the hypothesis that crowdsourcing could be used in residency training which could potentially provide a more objective appraisal process than the one where mentors who are invested in the trainee's advancement are also the ones determining if they are meeting the advancement benchmarks [22]. Three residents or differing post-graduate years and two expert robotic faculty performed a video-captured dry-lab robotic-assisted suturing task. These brief videos were posted to the Turker crowdsourcing platform and distributed to expert surgeons to rate using the abbreviated GEARS tool. Just as in the previous study, the average scores from the crowds and experts correlated well ($R = 0.91$). Another observation not predicted by the group was that one of the senior residents for this particular suturing task outscored one of the faculty members. Both the expert raters and the crowdworkers "saw" this. One could envision that if the raters were not blinded to the performers' expertise level – resident vs. faculty – the scores might have been different. However, in the CSATS process, reviewers are blinded to the reviewees' identities and demographics. In that same study, the authors also tested whether the skill advancement of a trainee could be detected after robotic skills instruction. An individual mid-level resident performed the robotic-assisted suturing task, and the video was immediately sent during that that simulation training session to the crowdworkers. Fifteen minutes were spent by an instructor training the trainee and then a subsequent criterion suturing performance was captured and sent to the crowdworkers to rate. Within 1 hour from the first performance, the crowdworkers had assessed both videos and had identified improvement in the performer pre- and post-instruction. What could not be determined was how many of the crowdworkers were the same from the one survey to the next as the identities of the crowdworkers cannot be elucidated through the crowdsourcing platform. Although a limitation, another study has shown that the crowdsourcing process is reliable irrespective of the time of day, days of the week the surveys are posted [23].

The ability to assess trainee skill remotely and through video review provides opportunities that transcend our country's borders. White et al. used CSATS to assess a group of surgery residents from Ethiopia performing open basic dry-lab surgical tasks. The ratings, again, were rapid and derived from Amazon.com crowdworkers [24].

Because the CSATS process can handle high throughput of videos, it promises to accelerate the validation of new training curricula. In a study sponsored by the American Urological Association in an effort to validate a new laparoscopic training curriculum, Kowalewski et al. applied CSATS to perform the reviews of numerous videos which may have otherwise required an unrealistic effort from expert raters. The Basic Laparoscopic Urologic Surgery (BLUS) Curriculum is a cognitive and psychomotor curriculum devoted to training basic laparoscopic skills in urologic residents across the United States [25, 26]. The parent AUA organization had amassed over 450 videos of BLUS performances which included suturing tasks, object transfer tasks, a pattern cutting task, and a laparoscopic vessel clip-applying task. These videos were aggregated from eight academic centers from residents and faculty. The AUA needed to their 5 expert surgeons to review all 450 plus videos to score them using the GOALS tool in order to validate that the psychomotor portion of the BLUS curriculum could discriminate levels of skill. The directors felt that the reviewer burden was insurmountable and hypothesized perhaps crowdsourcing could be employed. In a pilot study, a subset of videos from the suturing and object transfer task (12 in each spanning the range of skill from novice to expert performer) were assessed by CSATS and by the AUA's expert review panel. The agreement for the suturing task was almost a perfect 1.0 [27]. From these results, the AUA felt that the CSATS methodology was reliable and decided to complete the validation process of the more than 400 remaining skills videos using crowdsourcing.

Relevant Surgery Skills Validation

In order for a new assessment process to yield value, it must be generalizable to surgical environments similar to human surgery. The previous validation centered in simulated dry-lab environments where the surgical video was highly structured and the content was standardized. In 2015, Holst et al. tested the hypothesis that crowdsourcing skills assessment could be used in a porcine robotic-assisted laparoscopic training environment. In their study, 12 surgeons of various skill levels performed a robotic-assisted intracorporeal urinary bladder suturing closure [22]. These videos were distributed to 50 crowdworkers and five expert surgeon raters to assess technique using the modified GEARS tool. The correlation between the two reviewer cohorts was Cronbach's alpha = 0.93. The crowdworkers did not require any training or orientation to the content they were reviewing and yet they scored like expert surgeon raters. It took less than 5 hours for all CSATS ratings to be completed.

These validation studies paved the way for the first study looking at whether crowdsourcing could be used to assess human surgery. Similar to the MBSC group, the Michigan Urologic Surgery Improvement Collaborative (MUSIC) seeks to share patient outcomes and clinical processes among a large group of urologists in the state of Michigan [19]. This collaborative, funded by the largest payer in the state, amasses outcomes data for prostate cancer patients. The collaborative's mission is to identify top performers and share their methods with the collaborative to raise the performance of all providers. One area this collaborative focuses on is the technical skills of providers when doing robotic-assisted laparoscopic prostatectomies (RALPs). The group had already established a process to capture, edit, and share video within the collaborative and they, much like the MBSC, thought that some sort of video review process might elevate the performance of all peers. While recruiting expert reviewers, they hypothesized that crowdworkers could also rate RALP performances. Twenty-two volunteers submitted video of their RALPs to the collaborative and had a blinded review using the GEARS tool completed by 25 peers and 680 crowdworkers. Ghani et al. demonstrated good correlation between the expert peer and crowdsourcing reviews ($r = 0.78$). Furthermore, review times paralleled previous CSATS studies with crowdworkers taking 38 hours to complete the reviews. The group made a relevant observation that the crowd workers and the expert peer raters agreed on which performances were the lowest five performances. As the collaborative tried to identify which surgeons might benefit from coaching, this group discussed that a rapid system to help identify coaching targets would be useful to improve outcomes. The same would be true in a training environment where any system that could rapidly triage trainees and alert mentors to those who need remediation, would enhance the acceleration of skills acquisition.

The MUSIC group then expanded this study and hypothesized that CSATS scores could predict patient outcomes. They captured and assessed surgical RAPL video from 29 surgeons and then tracked the patient outcomes for all prostatectomy patients by those surgeons for a year. A total of 2256 patients were included in the outcomes analysis [28]. Ghani et al. observed correlations between key clinical outcomes and the CSATS scores. The complication rates were higher among patients operated on by surgeons in the lowest quartile of CSATS scores compared to the top quartile. Furthermore, the rate of urethral catheter re-insertion after removal post-prostatectomy (as potential sign of a technical error at the urethrovesical anastomosis) was significantly higher among the bottom quartile performing surgeons based of CSATS scores. This was the first demonstration that crowdworkers' assessments could predict patient outcomes.

Surgery aptitude is not only about the ability of someone to suture tissues. Senior educators might suggest that exposing the target areas in surgery represent one of the critical steps in any surgery. Good exposure sets up a case for optimal performance. To test whether non-medically trained crowdworkers could discriminate the ability of a surgeon to expose a surgical field well, Powers et al. captured video from trainees and faculty doing robotic-assisted nephrectomies [29]. They created a survey tool adapted from GEARS and included a question about the adequacy of exposure of the renal hilum. This is a key step before controlling the blood supply to the kidney. In their study, they showed excellent agreement between crowd scores and expert reviewer scores. This was the first evidence of crowdworkers being able to assess a higher order step in a surgery beyond basic suturing.

Similar to the Powers et al. study, Deal et al. took the exposure question one step further and hypothesized that crowds could be trained to identify whether surgical decision-making or judgment was adequate [30]. In their study, videos from practicing general surgeons performing laparoscopic cholecystectomies were captured. Videos were edited down to the portion of the video where the Critical View of Safety (CVS) was identified. The CVS is the identification of the structures that make up the Triangle of Calot. Errant ligation of the common bile duct is a catastrophic complication during a laparoscopic cholecystectomy, and the American College of Surgery suggests all surgeons identify the CVS before clipping and ligation to reduce the chance of common bile duct injury [30]. Deal et al. used an assessment tool that qualifies the degree to which the CVS is adequately visualized. Expert surgeons used this tool and the Global Objective Assessment of Laparoscopic Skills (GOALS) to assess technique and the CVS survey tool. Crowdworkers also received both tools except the crowdworkers were first exposed to a tutorial detailing the CVS and the tool. The results showed that crowdworkers, after minimal training, could assess surgical judgment just as expert surgeon reviewers with CVS survey tool correlations of 0.89. The crowds also agreed with expert reviewers for technical skills with GOALS scores for 40 videos assessed.

Barriers to Adoption of a CSATS Methodology to Robotic Microsurgical Procedures in Plastic Surgery

When trying to advance the fields of plastic and reconstructive surgery, it is sometimes important to pivot one's gaze outside of the field and look at developments within other surgical subspecialties. As we have seen from the discussion of the development of CSATS, there currently exists timely and cost-effective methods to analyze the performance of robotic and laparoscopic procedures. These assessments are capable of stratifying surgeons according to technical skill and providing educational feedback to the operator in a timely and cost-effective manner. The benefits to patient care and our nation's system of surgical education is potentially substantial. The system can in theory be applied to any type of surgery whose performance can be captured on video. So what are the barriers to the adoption of such a system within plastic and reconstructive surgery?

It is worth noting that many of the metrics developed in OSATS, and deployed in the CSATS method, could be applied to plastic surgery procedures. The metrics that are evaluated using the OSATS criteria are factors that are capable of being analyzed in any surgical procedure where tissue is manipulated (i.e., hemostasis, tissue handling) – they are not unique to plastic surgical procedures. In fact, similar validated methods of evaluation have already been introduced to analyze robotic microsurgical procedures [31]. While it is true that as surgery becomes increasingly subject to objective and timely evaluation, the fidelity of these validated systems will likely increase. For example, assessment modules that track individual procedures (i.e., pedicled flap creation) or particular techniques (i.e., microsurgical anastomosis) could be created to track these procedural elements more effectively. Once these systems of evaluation are created, they could be easily deployed using a crowd-sourced methodology such as that developed by CSATS. In this respect, it is important to see the crowd-sourced methodology for what it is – *an efficient aggregator of human attention capable of making discerning evaluations of nearly any human activity*. As of this writing, no machine learning platform can provide the same fidelity or accuracy with respect to the evaluation of surgical performance. The authors recognize that this is likely only a temporary state of affairs.

There also exist technical factors that make open field surgery more difficult to analyze. The particular view provided by the camera in laparoscopic and robotic procedures works particularly well in blinding the observer to the operator and providing a standardized view for video analysis. Open field surgery is a process that is more likely to produce variability in video or photographic reproduction. As an example, the video that is generally captured during open field surgery (with the operator wearing a surgical headlight or loupe-mounted camera) is likely to include variable ratios in the size of the surgical field or include elements that might bias evaluators, such as the appearance of their extremities. Furthermore, variability in lighting and image capture are obviously more problematic. That being said, individual elements of surgical performance, for example microsurgical anastomosis, lend themselves particularly well to these situations – the view of the operating microscope being analogous to the endoscope in the standardization of the field of view. *Furthermore, it is important to recognize that none of the problems are insurmountable.* As previously discussed, crowd workers have proved capable of making valid discriminations regarding complex surgical tasks such as that of providing exposure – not merely the focused analysis of tissue manipulation. For instance, software could very well be created that analyzes surgical video postoperatively (perhaps by placing fiducials to frame the operative field) and provides experts or crowdworkers with an appropriately standardized view of the operative maneuvers performed during open surgery. Systems could also be developed to greatly diminish the variability in quality of operative video produced by open-field cameras.

Conclusion

This chapter discussed the creation and application of a novel crowd-sourced platform for the evaluation of surgical skill – CSATS. The platform, based on the validated assessments of lay crowdworkers, provides a timely and cost-effective method to assess surgical skill. The platform has been successfully applied to several procedures and offers a promising method of skills assessment for numerous procedures performed in both laparoscopic or robotic-assisted settings and in a wide variety of surgical disciplines. This tool seems primed for evaluation of robotic microsurgical skill evaluation for both training and credentialing.

Disclosure   Authors Lendvay and Smartt were prior shareholders in CSATS Inc.

References

1. Birkmeyer JD, et al. Surgical skill and complication rates after bariatric surgery. N Engl J Med. 2013;369(15):1434–42.
2. Donaldson MS. An overview of to err is human: re-emphasizing the message of patient safety. In: Hughes RG, editor. Patient safety and quality: an evidence-based handbook for nurses. Rockville: Agency for Healthcare Research and Quality; 2008.
3. Weiser TG, et al. An estimation of the global volume of surgery: a modelling strategy based on available data. Lancet. 2008;372(9633):139–44.
4. American College of Surgeons. Health Policy Research Institute; Association of American Medical Colleges. The surgery workforce in the United States: profile and recent trends. Washington, DC: Association of American Medical Colleges; 2010.
5. Nasca TJ, et al. The next GME accreditation system--rationale and benefits. N Engl J Med. 2012;366(11):1051–6.
6. Sosa JA, et al. The importance of surgeon experience for clinical and economic outcomes from thyroidectomy. Ann Surg. 1998;228(3):320–30.
7. Schmidt CM, et al. Effect of hospital volume, surgeon experience, and surgeon volume on patient outcomes after pancreaticoduodenectomy: a single-institution experience. Arch Surg. 2010;145(7):634–40.
8. Mendivil A, Holloway RW, Boggess JF. Emergence of robotic assisted surgery in gynecologic oncology: American perspective. Gynecol Oncol. 2009;114(2 Suppl):S24–31.
9. Zorn KC, et al. Training, credentialing, proctoring and medicolegal risks of robotic urological surgery: recommendations of the society of urologic robotic surgeons. J Urol. 2009;182(3):1126–32.
10. Matsuda T, et al. The endoscopic surgical skill qualification system in urological laparoscopy: a novel system in Japan. J Urol. 2006;176(5):2168–72; discussion 2172.
11. Matsuda T, et al. Reliability of laparoscopic skills assessment on video: 8-year results of the endoscopic surgical skill qualification system in Japan. J Endourol. 2014;28(11):1374–8.
12. Martin JA, et al. Objective structured assessment of technical skill (OSATS) for surgical residents. Br J Surg. 1997;84(2):273–8.

13. Hogg ME, et al. Grading of surgeon technical performance predicts postoperative pancreatic fistula for pancreaticoduodenectomy independent of patient-related variables. Ann Surg. 2016;264(3):482–91.
14. Goh AC, et al. Global evaluative assessment of robotic skills: validation of a clinical assessment tool to measure robotic surgical skills. J Urol. 2012;187(1):247–52.
15. Vassiliou MC, et al. A global assessment tool for evaluation of intraoperative laparoscopic skills. Am J Surg. 2005;190(1):107–13.
16. Ezra DG, et al. Skills acquisition and assessment after a microsurgical skills course for ophthalmology residents. Ophthalmology. 2009;116(2):257–62.
17. Kurashima Y, et al. A tool for training and evaluation of laparoscopic inguinal hernia repair: the Global Operative Assessment of Laparoscopic Skills-Groin Hernia (GOALS-GH). Am J Surg. 2011;201(1):54–61.
18. Korndorffer JR Jr, et al. Simulator training for laparoscopic suturing using performance goals translates to the operating room. J Am Coll Surg. 2005;201(1):23–9.
19. Ghani KR, et al. Measuring to improve: peer and crowd-sourced assessments of technical skill with robot-assisted radical prostatectomy. Eur Urol. 2016;69(4):547–50.
20. Chen C, et al. Crowd-sourced assessment of technical skills: a novel method to evaluate surgical performance. J Surg Res. 2014;187(1):65–71.
21. White LW, et al. Crowd-sourced assessment of technical skill: a valid method for discriminating basic robotic surgery skills. J Endourol. 2015;29(11):1295–301.
22. Holst D, et al. Crowd-sourced assessment of technical skills: differentiating animate surgical skill through the wisdom of crowds. J Endourol. 2015;29(10):1183–8.
23. Lendvay TS, Ghani KR, Peabody JO, Linsell S, Miller DC, Comstock B. Is crowdsourcing surgical skill assessment reliable? An analysis of robotic prostatectomies. J Urol. 2017;197(4):E890–1.
24. White LW, Lendvay TS, Holst D, Borbely Y, Bekele A, Wright A. Using crowd-assessment to support surgical training in the developing world. J Am Coll Surg. 2014;219(4):e40.
25. Sweet RM, et al. Introduction and validation of the American Urological Association Basic Laparoscopic Urologic Surgery skills curriculum. J Endourol. 2012;26(2):190–6.
26. Kowalewski TM, et al. Validation of the AUA BLUS tasks. J Urol. 2016;195(4 Pt 1):998–1005.
27. Kowalewski TM, et al. Crowd-sourced assessment of technical skills for validation of basic laparoscopic urologic skills tasks. J Urol. 2016;195(6):1859–65.
28. Ghani KR, Comstock B, Miller DC, Dunn RL, Kim T, Linsell S, Lane BR, Sarle R, Lendvay T, Montie J, Peabody JO. Technical skill assessment of surgeons performing robot-assisted radical prostatectomy: relationship between crowdsourced review and patient outcomes. J Urol. 2017;197(4):e609.
29. Powers MK, et al. Crowdsourcing assessment of surgeon dissection of renal artery and vein during robotic partial nephrectomy: a novel approach for quantitative assessment of surgical performance. J Endourol. 2016;30(4):447–52.
30. Deal SB, et al. Evaluation of crowd-sourced assessment of the critical view of safety in laparoscopic cholecystectomy. Surg Endosc. 2017;31(12):5094–100.
31. Alrasheed T, et al. Robotic microsurgery: validating an assessment tool and plotting the learning curve. Plast Reconstr Surg. 2014;134(4):794–803.

Part II

Clinical Applications

Robotic Harvest of the Rectus Abdominis Muscle

Chad M. Bailey, Geraldine T. Klein, John C. Pedersen, Louis L. Pisters, and Jesse C. Selber

Introduction

The rectus abdominis muscle has been a staple of reconstructive surgery for decades. Its reliable anatomy, muscle bulk, pedicle length, and relative ease of harvest account for its multiple indications and uses. Whether addressing chest wall, breast or pelvic defects with a pedicled flap, or distant defects of the head and neck or extremities with free tissue transfer, the rectus is a reliable source of well-vascularized tissue with which to cover wounds, obliterate dead space, and fill large defects. With standard harvest techniques, a midline laparotomy or paramedian incision directly over one muscle belly is necessary for exposure and harvest. This requires a large incision in the anterior rectus fascia for exposure. As the anterior rectus is the strength layer of the abdominal wall, violation of it can lead to bulging (laxity in the anterior abdominal wall) or herniation of the intra-abdominal contents. In a patient that does not require a laparotomy, this adds significant morbidity.

Electronic Supplementary Material The online version of this chapter (https://doi.org/10.1007/978-3-030-74244-7_3) contains supplementary material, which is available to authorized users.

C. M. Bailey
Division of Proliance Surgeons, Plastic & Reconstructive Surgeons, Renton, WA, USA

G. T. Klein
Eisenhower Medical Association, Rancho Mirage, CA, USA

J. C. Pedersen
Plastic Surgery, Cleveland Clinic, Akron, OH, USA

L. L. Pisters
The University of Texas MD Anderson Cancer Center, Houston, TX, USA

J. C. Selber (✉)
Department of Plastic Surgery, MD Anderson Cancer Center, Houston, TX, USA
e-mail: jcselber@mdanderson.org

© Springer Nature Switzerland AG 2021
J. C. Selber (ed.), *Robotics in Plastic and Reconstructive Surgery*,
https://doi.org/10.1007/978-3-030-74244-7_3

When a rectus is required for pelvic reconstruction, particularly after a robotic-assisted procedure has been performed, robotic-assisted techniques of harvest are clearly favored [1, 2]. Robotic-assisted harvest in these scenarios eliminates the need for a laparotomy, as well as an anterior rectus fascia incision, repair of which frequently can call for the use of prosthetic mesh. A robotic-assisted rectus flap may also improve operative efficiency as side docking of the patient cart allows the graft to be harvested simultaneously to another surgical team performing part of a pelvic dissection from a perineal or transvaginal approach. When free transfer of the rectus abdominis is required, robotic-assisted harvest offers a less invasive approach, minimizing postoperative recovery time, abdominal bulging, and hernias.

There are unique aspects of the rectus abdominis muscle that lend it to robotic-assisted harvest. These include its intra-abdominal location allowing for clear posterior visualization of the flap and pedicle; a long and frequently visible pedicle when viewed from inside the abdomen, relative safety of "blind" dissection around the medial, anterior, and lateral aspects of the rectus muscle; relative pliability allowing for extraction through a small midline incision when needed; and lack of need for large amounts of clip ligation of perforating side-branches.

Flap Anatomy

The rectus abdominis muscle is a long, relatively thin muscle running longitudinally along the anterior abdominal wall. The muscle is enveloped in a fascial sheath throughout most of its length. The anterior rectus sheath drapes the entire anterior surface of the muscle, while the posterior rectus sheath supports the posterior surface of the muscle from the lower costal cartilage to the arcuate line, approximately one-third the distance from the umbilicus to the pubic symphysis. The posterior portion of the muscle inferior to the arcuate line is covered by a thin layer of transversalis fascia as well as parietal peritoneum, neither of which provide mechanical strength. The muscle is also divided by three to four transverse tendinous inscriptions, which shorten the moment arm of force for each segment, allowing the muscle to distribute force differentially over its distance.

The muscle originates from the pubic crest and symphysis and inserts into the costal cartilage of the 5th–7th ribs (posterior to the pectoralis major). Motor branches supply the rectus from the 7th–12th intercostal nerves, entering the muscle on its lateral surface and travelling infero-medially after entering the muscle [3].

The rectus abdominis functions as a trunk flexor, specifically flexing the vertebral column. Removal of one or both recti has been performed, most often for breast reconstruction. This results in minimal to moderate functional morbidity (the overwhelming majority of patients return to their baseline preoperative activity level) due to the ability of the remaining trunk musculature to compensate for the absence of the rectus, although long-term functional limitations can remain [4, 5].

The rectus abdominis muscle is classically described as having a "dual" blood supply (Mathes and Nahai type III), but in reality is served by a dominant blood supply from the deep inferior epigastric artery, with a less dominant contribution from the superior epigastric artery that can be augmented with deep inferior epigastric artery ligation [6]. The rectus abdominis flap, when used for pelvic reconstruction or free tissue transfer, is isolated on the deep inferior epigastric artery and vein. When used for lower chest wall reconstruction, the rectus can be based on the superior epigastric artery without need for the delay or venous or arterial augmentation.

From the external iliac artery and vein, the deep inferior epigastric pedicle reliably runs underneath posterior to the rectus abdominis muscle for several centimeters until entering the muscle just inferior to the arcuate line and branching in one of four described patterns either just before entering or within the muscle [7].

Indications and Contraindications for Robotic-Assisted Rectus Harvest

The indications for a robotic-assisted rectus abdominis harvest are nearly any that call for use of the rectus abdominis muscle for reconstruction, and do not require additional skin and subcutaneous fat. Contraindications to robotic-assisted rectus abdominis harvest include evidence of a frozen abdomen, multiple previous intra-abdominal procedures, or presence of a large ventral hernia that requires open repair.

Advantages

The advantages of robot-assisted rectus harvest include eliminating the need for a laparotomy and anterior rectus sheath incision, as well as reducing the need for mesh reinforcement and an external drain. Postoperative restrictions are also minimal and do not typically include the use of an abdominal binder. Postoperative hernia and bulge rates are theoretically reduced.

Disadvantages

The main disadvantage of the robot-assisted technique is the time and effort required of the surgeon to establish and credential for the use of the robot, and this has been described in detail [8]. Additional disadvantages include the additional cost and manpower required to operate the surgical robot (these may be offset by decreased postoperative length of stay), surgical robot availability, and obtaining adequate training to use the surgical robot. It should be noted, however, that the base charge for a robotic room facility fee is approximately double that of a regular OR, so the facility fee makes the institution money during a robotic case. Additional disadvantages include the limitations of use in patients with multiple previous abdominal operations, including the potential need for general surgery assistance entering the abdomen, the potential for intra-abdominal organ injury, and potential port site bleeding. The inherent risks of laparoscopic surgery also exist, including the potential for uncontrollable intra-abdominal bleeding requiring conversion to an open procedure. None of these issues have transpired in our series.

Surgical Technique

Patient Positioning

The patient can be placed supine or in a low lithotomy position in stirrups, depending on whether a simultaneous pelvic procedure is being performed. Preparation and draping should expose the entire abdominal wall and flank, from the midsternum to the pubic symphysis. If pelvic extirpation is being performed, position changes are typically not required. Patient immobilization to the OR table is key, as extremes of bed positioning may be required to maneuver intra-abdominal contents to improve ease of dissection. Tucking of the arms is generally recommended; however, if anesthesia requests access, the arm contralateral to the rectus being harvested is most conveniently abducted. Attention to the positioning of the contralateral arm relative to the robotic arms is necessary and will be covered later in this chapter.

Docking and Port Placement

Of utmost importance in a robotic-assisted rectus abdominis harvest is port location and arm placement. The time and thought devoted to these critical steps are well worth the effort and will dictate the ease (or difficulty) of the case. In the case of a previously performed robotic procedure, the surgeon should never hesitate to place new ports. Compromise on the approach to the rectus due to poor port placement will ultimately cause a surgical delay or difficulty in execution.

We first mark the costal margin and the superior iliac spine, connecting the two with a line along the anterior axillary line for reference. The authors' preferred technique is to place 8 mm intraperitoneal robotic ports oriented obliquely from the anterior superior iliac spine (most lateral) to the subcostal margin (most medial). Ports are placed contralateral to the planned rectus harvest, with the robot boom placed ipsilateral to the rectus being harvest. An Ultra Veress Needle (Ethicon, Somerville, NJ) is used to enter the peritoneum when a simultaneous intra-abdominal procedure is not being performed (Fig. 3.1). Insufflation is obtained and the camera (central) port is then placed just cephalad to the level of the umbilicus and 2–4 cm lateral to the semi-lunar line, followed by examination of the intra-abdominal contents with the laparoscopic camera. This step is easily circumvented in the case of a simultaneous intra-abdominal procedure (Fig. 3.2), as insufflation has already been achieved and the existing ports can be used to introduce a laparoscopic camera to facilitate new port placement. The remaining instrument ports are then placed under direct vision, generally favoring as lateral and posterior placement as the colon will allow for the most caudal port (typically just superior to the ASIS, Figs. 3.3 and

Fig. 3.1 Intraperitoneal
access. Veress needle
(Ethicon, Somerville, NJ)
is used to enter the
peritoneum and obtain the
pneumoperitoneum
following standard
pressure guidelines when a
simultaneous pelvic or
abdominal ablative
procedure is not being
performed

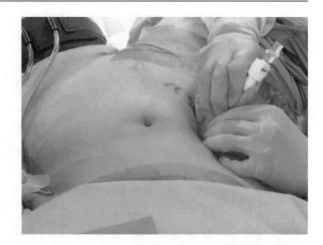

Fig. 3.2 Port placement 1.
Lateral view of typical port
placement for a robotic
rectus. Three ports are
placed, one at the costal
margin, one above the iliac
crest, and one between the
two. The camera port is the
central port and the other
two are for
instrumentation. Ports are
placed as lateral as
possible without
encroaching on abdominal
viscera

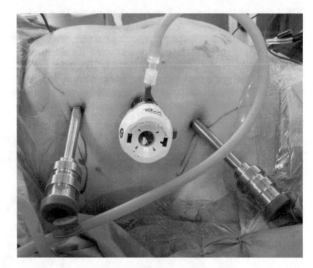

3.4). The most cephalad port is then placed just caudal to the subcostal margin within the semi-lunar line (which is more medial at this level). Simply put, the three ports should frequently be as lateral as possible on the contralateral side, and evenly split the distance between the ilium and the costal margin. We have found this port orientation allows for ample range of motion when approaching the contralateral deep inferior epigastric pedicle, which is always significantly caudal to the port placement. It is important to note that in this arrangement instrument and camera ports are interchangeable when using the Xi system, allowing for instrument and camera exchanges during extremes of dissection (typically needed for the most cranial and caudal portions of dissection).

After port placement, the surgical robot ("patient cart") is then stationed perpendicular to the patient, on the ipsilateral side of the rectus muscle being harvested, until a 90° angle can be achieved with the camera arm (either arm 2 or 3 with the Xi

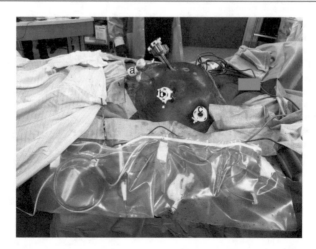

Fig. 3.3 Port placement 2. Three ports to be used for rectus harvest. In this image prior to exchange to robotic ports, the location of the right lateral ports (a, b, and c) are near ideal for a left rectus abdominis harvest. *a*, most superomedial port, just below the costal cartilage, typically near the semi-lunar line. *b*, middle port, typically near the anterior axillary line; this is the typical location of the camera when using either the Si or Xi systems. *c*, inferolateral port, typically used for the curved monopolar scissors; this port lies near the mid-axillary line (lateral placement is limited by intra-abdominal contents) and just cephalad to the anterior superior iliac spine. *, umbilical port, when present, is ideal to monitor port placement with the laparoscopic camera

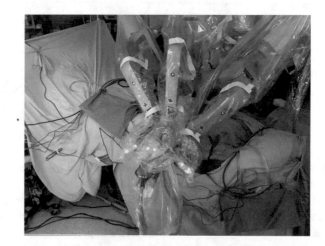

Fig. 3.4 Robotic arm positioning for the da Vinci. The patient cart is stationed ipsilateral to the rectus being dissected and perpendicular to the patient. The camera arm is flexed 90° at the elbow. Maximizing distance between patient clearance joints is essential. Instrument arm elbows are placed akimbo to the camera arm to minimize interference. Ports are placed contralateral to the rectus being harvested

Fig. 3.5 Case example. After having an exposed and infected arthroplasty endoprosthesis, this patient received a robotically harvested rectus muscle to cover the prosthesis. The muscle can be extracted using a small incision in the pubic hairline or through a 12 mm port using a laparoscopic retrieval bag

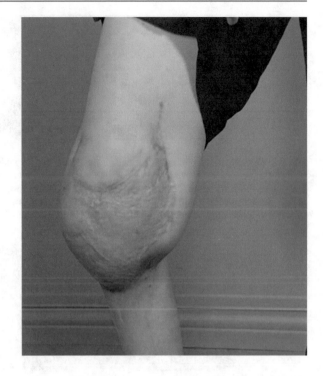

system). Initial basic arm positioning is achieved selecting the "lower abdominal" setting on the patient cart touch pad. The central column of the surgical robot is typically positioned at the level of the umbilicus, and the camera port is docked first. If using the Xi system, we have found the targeting feature to be of some benefit [9], though final manipulation of the instrument arms is always necessary to minimize conflict with the camera arm. Maximizing distance between patient clearance joints after precise port placement is essential, and this is accomplished prior to instrument introduction after camera placement using the patient clearance buttons on the instrument arm [10]. Once arm positioning is satisfactory (Fig. 3.5), the unused arm (arm 3 with the Si, 1 or 4 with Xi) is stowed (collapsed, rotated away nearest the column, and lifted) and the instrument arms are docked and the instruments placed under direct visualization from the endoscopic camera [11].

Instruments and Positioning

The senior author uses the da Vinci Si and Xi robotic surgical systems (Intuitive Surgical, Sunnyvale, CA) depending on institutional availability. The Xi is optimal, particularly when redocking is necessary, since the base of the robot does not need to be moved. The instruments of choice include an 8 mm 30° endoscope (available with the Xi), monopolar curved scissors in the dominant arm (*HotShears*™, Intuitive Surgical, Sunnyvale, CA), and fenestrated bipolar forceps in the non-dominant arm.

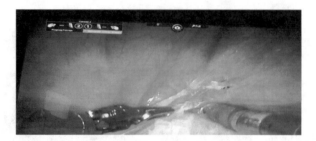

Fig. 3.6 Opening of the peritoneum and identification of the deep inferior epigastric pedicle. The pedicle can be seen in this video as a blue hue from the top right of the screen down through the opening of the peritoneum. The non-dominant hand is critical to opening of the parietal perito-neum. Tension on the peritoneum allows for the use of monopolar cautery (curved monopolar scissors) to incise the peritoneum and identification of the pedicle

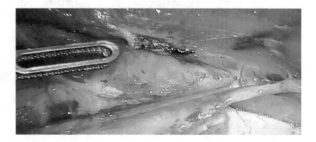

Fig. 3.7 Perforator dissection technique. Proximal perforator entering the rectus directly from the pedicle. The perforator is isolated via blunt dissection. Once isolated, the perforator is cauterized with bipolar cautery and ligated sharply with the monopolar curved scissors

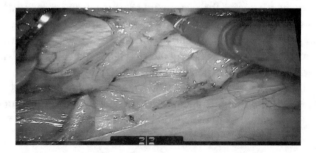

Fig. 3.8 Pedicle dissection techniques (timelapse). A combination of blunt tension (with non-dominant hand fenestrated bipolar forceps) and judicious monopolar cautery with dominant hand curved monopolar forceps allows for a dissection that reveals perforators of significance and con-trols minor bleeding from the peri-pedicle fat

When using the Si, a 12 mm port must be placed due to the caliber of the camera (we prefer to put this in the middle port), and "port hopping" is limited/impossible unless larger ports are placed throughout [12]. The majority of the dissection is performed with the monopolar curved scissors, including small perforator cauter-ization, with the fenestrated bipolar forceps serving to provide tension (Figs. 3.6,

3.7, and 3.8). Additional instruments used include the large clip applier (Weck *Hemo-lock*® clips, Intuitive Surgical, Sunnyvale, CA) for pedicle ligation when a free flap is performed, and needle drivers for posterior rectus sheath closure.

Cautery is typically set at 25/25 (cut/coag) when using the Si system, or 5/5 when using the ERBE VIO dV® generator with the Xi system. Insufflation is typically set at 15 mmHg, with a flow rate of 3 L/min. The patient is placed in moderate to extreme Trendelenburg as well as rotation contralateral to the muscle being harvested to mobilize the intra-abdominal contents opposite of the dissection. We typically reduce intra-abdominal insufflation at the time of posterior rectus sheath closure to 10–12 mmHg to reduce tension.

Flap Harvest

In cases where concomitant urinary diversion is being performed, the left rectus muscle is preferentially harvested to allow maturation of the ileal conduit through the right-sided rectus muscle. With the pedicle typically visible, either directly or by pulsation through the peri-pedicle fat, we begin dissection immediately over the pedicle with a combination of blunt dissection, sharp dissection, and cautery (Fig. 3.6). Careful attention is paid to tension on the peritoneum, elevating the peritoneum off of the pedicle, allowing for more aggressive and calculated dissection away from the pedicle. Once the peritoneum is incised and the pre-peritoneal space is entered, dissection is continued in a similar manner, with care to further open the peritoneum cranially and caudally to maximize exposure safely. The peritoneal incision is then carried medially so that the medial edge of the muscle can be identified without obstruction of the view by the peritoneal flap. This will create one single peritoneal flap that can be sutured closed after flap harvest. If a significant amount of peri-pedicle fat is present, this does not require extensive dissection, as long as the pedicle is visualized, until the vessels require isolation. Blunt dissection is key to pedicle isolation in these scenarios, and many times this can be aided with the use of the Maryland Bipolar Forceps to improve the ease of this dissection.

Pedicle dissection is continued cranially, with assistance from the assistant hand (fenestrated bipolar forceps) pushing (not grasping) the pedicle posteriorly to provide tension the way a vessel loop might be used. The entire length of the pedicle must be continually visualized due to the lack of tactile feedback afforded by the surgical robot. If perforators are encountered that require ligation, these can be safely ligated with bipolar electrocautery (Fig. 3.7). This must be carried out with caution and with extreme precision. An alternative method would be to employ the small clip applier (Weck Horizon small-wide titanium clips). When several perforators are present, clip ligation can be significantly time consuming, as each individual clip requires reloading, comprising of complete instrument removal and replacement. If perforators are small and can be isolated well away from the pedicle, bipolar cautery is preferred, emphasizing the usefulness of the fenestrated bipolar forceps as a grasper and a tool for cauterization. If there are a number of larger branches, they can be dissected and then divided with the Vessel Sealer, a device much like the Ligasure.

Once the pedicle enters the rectus abdominis, dissection is then focused on isolation of the muscle, which is aided by opening of the posterior rectus sheath longitudinally along its medial aspect. This is incised with cautery (monopolar curved scissors) to limit bleeding. This dissection is inherently safe as the pedicle enters the muscle laterally. Pharmacologic paralysis is helpful at this point to avoid muscle contraction, although direct stimulation of the muscle with cautery is common. The dissection is significantly aided by teasing and pushing of the rectus with the non-dominant hand along the medial edge of the muscle, retracting the muscle posteriorly. Anterior dissection is carried laterally, until the most lateral aspect of the muscle is encountered along the semi-lunar line. Dissection off the posterior rectus sheath can be performed as well from this position, or a portion of the posterior rectus sheath can be taken with the flap.

As the surgeon dissects the rectus anteriorly, inscriptions can be a nuisance. We have found that these are best handled by maximizing the dissection on either side of the inscription before addressing the inscription itself, (when possible) and dividing the inscriptions with a combination of sharp dissection and electrocauterization, as in an open dissection. The monopolar curved scissors offer a combination of features that allow the surgeon to accomplish this with minimal violation of the anterior rectus sheath or disruption of muscle continuity. Scant and interrupted violation of the anterior rectus sheath should not be viewed as a significant problem, as the posterior rectus sheath will typically be closed at the end of the procedure. However, any large rents should be closed with interrupted suture.

Once the muscle is isolated cranially, attention turns to transection. This is performed with electrocautery with the monopolar curved scissors/*HotShears*™. We do not attempt to isolate or clip ligate the superior epigastric vessels, as cautery is safe and less time consuming. An attempt at isolation of these vessels also creates the potential for uncontrolled bleeding, which can be significant.

Once the muscle is transected cranially, final freeing of the muscle from the rectus sheath with blunt, sharp, and cautery dissection is accomplished, completely liberating the muscle from the surrounding sheath. When a pedicled flap is needed, depending on the pelvic defect, caudal dissection is carried down as far as required. The flap can be disinserted from the pubis and islandized on the pedicle for greater mobility in the pelvis or left attached, according to surgeon preference. If caudal rectus transection is required to increase reach, this is performed in a similar manner the cranial release.

If free tissue transfer is planned, caudal transection of both the muscular attachment to the pubis and pedicle control and ligation are required. We attempt to achieve the maximum pedicle length for all cases. Once the vessels are isolated at their most caudal point, ligation is accomplished with a clip applier (Weck *Hem-o-lock*® clips, Fig. 3.9); 2–3 clips are typically used to ensure hemostasis.

Once free, the flap can be delivered in one of the two ways. When a 12 mm port is present, we prefer to deliver the flap via a laparoscopic retrieval sac (Anchor Products, Addison, IL). When 8 mm ports are used exclusively, a 2 cm hairline incision can be made over the pubis to deliver the tissue directly.

At this time, our preference is to primarily close the posterior rectus sheath, though this has been handled in a variety of ways. No one closure technique has

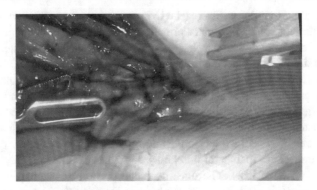

Fig. 3.9 Clip ligation of the deep inferior epigastric pedicle to the rectus abdominis flap. Once the pedicle and the flap have been completely isolated, clip ligation is performed with the Weck *Hemo-lock*® clip (Intuitive Surgical, Sunnyvale, CA). We routinely use 2–3 clips to ensure an absence of bleeding after ligation, which could be catastrophic and require exploratory laparotomy

been found to be superior to the other. We prefer running closure with a barbed suture, but the posterior rectus sheath has also been left open or reinforced with laparoscopic mesh in the past. We do not place a drain for rectus harvest alone, and, though one may be required after a simultaneous intra-abdominal procedure, drainage for the rectus dissection in these scenarios is not required. Instruments are exchanged to needle holders for both arms. A 2-0 V-loc suture (Medtronic, Minneapolis, MN) is introduced into the abdomen, and, after looping the suture in the posterior peritoneum or rectus sheath, the posterior rectus sheath and the peritoneum are closed primarily in a running fashion; this can be limited when a portion of the posterior rectus sheath has been removed with the flap. The maximum portion of posterior rectus sheath that can primarily closed is deemed satisfactory in these scenarios. Decreasing insufflation to 10–12 mmHg aids significantly to ease closure, but the surgeon may be limited by intra-abdominal contents and patient habitus. The suture is not knotted, but rather run back in the opposite direction of closure for one to three passes prior to transection with the needle drivers. Caudally, a bite of the anterior sheath is taken and incorporated into the closure to prevent herniation of abdominal contents into the empty rectus sheath.

Closure of the 8 mm ports is accomplished with simple dermal and epidermal sutures. Direct visualization of port removal should be performed when possible to ensure no port site bleeding. When a 12 mm port is placed or when a separate fascial incision is made to deliver the flap, the fascia can be closed in standard fashion. The entire procedure from docking to closure takes around 1 hour [1].

Urologic Indications and Pelvic Inset (for Pedicled Flaps)

The robot-assisted rectus flap harvest is of specific interest to the pelvic surgeon, particularly in urologic or urogynecologic surgeries. In the setting of robot-assisted abdominal or pelvic surgery, the pedicled rectus flap lays directly adjacent to the surgical field and can be easily reached via the same approach. A robotic rectus abdominis harvest can be easily performed as an adjunct to a robotic pelvic case in which the first steps of the flap harvest have already been completed including insufflation, initial port placement, and any necessary adhesiolysis. Other than the usual care to avoid injury to the inferior epigastric vessels during port placement, no specific precautions need to be met by the urologic/pelvic surgery team. For most robotic pelvic surgery, repositioning of only two robotic ports is needed to facilitate robotic-assisted rectus flap harvest. The skin of the prior port sites ipsilateral to the harvest site can be closed with a simple interrupted stitch to avoid loss of the pneumoperitoneum. These ipsilateral ports may be replaced following elevation of the rectus flap for pelvic inset. The most cephalad portion of the flap is commonly secured in the pelvis with dissolvable sutures in the most dependent portion of the pelvis. For patients requiring robotic salvage prostatectomy, cystectomy and ileal diversion, this is one of the only solutions that obliterates pelvic deadspace and prevents a urethrocutaneous fisutla.

In comparison to other flaps commonly used by pelvic surgeons to close dead space or assist with healing in the pelvis such as omental, peritoneal, gracilis, or Martius flaps, the robotic rectus flap has a robust blood supply and can easily reach anywhere in the pelvis. The advent of this minimally invasive harvesting approach expands and immensely improves upon future application.

In our practice, rectus flaps have been used in the setting of salvage cystectomies in previously radiated patients or in salvage prostatectomies with multiple risk factors for later fistula formation. Multiple other indications exist and call for this procedure, including in the repair of vesicovaginal fistulas, rectourethral fistulas, and in complex cases that may allow repair and bladder preservation in patients that would have previously been best managed non-operatively.

Postoperative Care

Postoperative restrictions and care are dictated by the additional procedures performed, whether an intra-abdominal extirpation or free tissue transfer. We do not use abdominal binders for robotic-assisted rectus harvest, nor do we have postoperative activity or weightbearing restrictions specific to the rectus harvest. Postoperative diet is directed by ileus (typically on a regular diet by postoperative day 1 if performing a rectus for free tissue transfer).

Outcomes

Pedersen, Song, and Selber have described the most robust series of robotic-assisted rectus flap harvests to date [1]. In their series, they reported complete flap survival (4 free, 6 pedicled) in all patients. Average time to set up the robot was 15 minutes (range 10–32 minutes), and the average harvest time was 45 minutes (range 31–126 minutes). No surgical complications were reported, and all flaps were viable following harvest. No procedures were converted to an open technique. To date, no long-term outcomes regarding abdominal morbidity have been described. Anecdotally, we have not witnessed abdominal hernias or bulging after robotic-assisted rectus harvest, no perceived weakness (by the patient), and no prolonged narcotic use due to the abdominal donor site.

Case Examples

Case 1 A 30-year-old female marathon runner presented for right lower extremity limb salvage. Her medical history was remarkable for reticular cell sarcoma of the right lower thigh that was treated with resection followed by chemotherapy and radiation therapy. She remained active, in spite of severe atrophy of the affected leg muscles. Because of worsening arthritis, she underwent a right knee arthroplasty. Two months postoperatively, the incision dehisced and she developed hardware-related infection. After washout and debridement, she underwent prosthesis exchange and negative-pressure wound therapy. Because her native musculature was atrophied and irradiated, there was no local muscle available for reconstruction. The decision was made to use a free rectus abdominis muscle free flap for limb salvage. A robotic muscle harvest was performed and the flap anastomosed end to side to the distal superficial femoral vessels, providing well-vascularized tissue over the exposed tendon and bone. The muscle was skin grafted and she went on to heal uneventfully (Fig. 3.10).

Case 2 A 62-year-old man presented with a history of high-risk prostate cancer. He received preoperative radiotherapy. Because his tumor was close to the rectum, plans were made for the patient to undergo radical robotic prostatectomy, possible robotic low anterior resection, and possible robotic rectus abdominis muscle flap for interposition between the coloanal anastomosis and urethrovesical anastomosis to prevent rectourethral fistula. During his prostatectomy, the rectum was injured

Fig. 3.10 Case 1. The donor site is shown for the robotic recuts is shown below. The scars are three small incisions on the contralateral side to the muscle being harvested. Incisional morbidity is very low, and there is no bulge appreciated

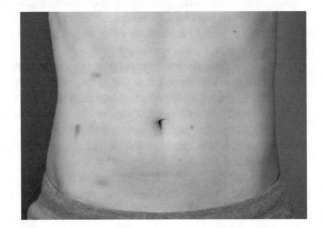

because of the proximity of the tumor, and a robotic imbricating repair was performed by a gastrointestinal surgeon. Port sites and robot position were changed, and a robotic rectus abdominis flap was performed. An umbilical hernia repair was also performed robotically using biologic mesh. The robot was re-docked to the prostate ports and the muscle was sutured to the pelvic floor between the rectum and the bladder. The urethrovesical anastomosis was then performed robotically and a temporary diverting ileostomy was created.

Pearls and Pitfalls

- *Port Placement and Robotic Arm Positioning*: Not paying careful attention to port placement and robotic arm positioning is the difference between a seemingly simple procedure, and one filled with hardship and headache. Careful attention to the anatomy, especially after placement of the camera port and prior to placing the instrument ports, is essential. Once docked, the robotic arms should be manipulated so that there is maximal space between individual arms and elbows while remaining within the "sweet spot" of each robot arm, as well as optimizing the upward "burp" on the ports to allow an optimal angle to access the anterior abdominal wall. Correction after dissection has begun is difficult and time intensive, and incorrect placement can ultimately limit the capabilities of the surgeon.
- *Monopolar Curved Scissors*/HotShears™: We have found the monopolar curved scissors are the most efficient for rectus dissection in the surgeon's dominant hand. This instrument allows the dissection to proceed swiftly and minimizes the need for instrument change.
- *Clip Ligation*: The rectus abdominis dissection, the deep inferior epigastric artery flap, and latissimus dorsi all lend themselves to robotic-assisted harvest in part due to the minimal need for clip ligation of side-branches. When needed, this is time consuming and requires instrument exchange. For the rectus abdominis dissection, the majority of small vessel branches can be successfully ligated with bipolar fenestrated forceps, and cranial flap transection can be successfully accomplished with monopolar cautery alone. We attempt to limit the use of clip ligation for pedicle transection only; however, a lap clip applier can be placed through any port when necessary.
- *Posterior Rectus Sheath*: Handling of the posterior rectus sheath after flap harvest is individual. We prefer to primarily close this with a barbed suture to eliminate knot tying and provide additional reinforcement to the abdominal wall. This closure is simple and only takes about 15 minutes. We have also left the posterior rectus sheath open, partially open, and have reinforced the posterior rectus sheath with laparoscopic hernia mesh. Handling of the posterior sheath is at the surgeon's discretion.
- *Pelvic Inset*: Though the urologic surgeons generally prefer to secure the rectus in the pelvis, the plastic surgeon can perform this step as well, quite easily. We place the flap in the pelvis and, if not performing the inset, always monitor this

step, pointing out the location of the pedicle frequently so the urologist or colorectal surgeon may avoid kinking, tension, or direct injury.

- *Postoperative Binder and Restrictions*: Postoperative care is minimal, and we do not routinely use abdominal binders or place drains for the rectus component of the operation. Similarly, the robotic-assisted rectus harvest places no additional restrictions on the patient beyond the limitations of lower extremity free tissue transfer or pelvic extirpation/exenteration.

References

1. Pedersen J, Song DH, Selber JC. Robotic, intraperitoneal harvest of the rectus abdominis muscle. Plast Reconstr Surg. 2014;134:1057–63.
2. Ibrahim A, Sarhane K, Pederson J, Selber J. Robotic harvest of the rectus abdominis muscle: principles and clinical applications. Semin Plast Surg. 2014;28:026–31.
3. Tessone A, Nava M, Blondeel P, Spano A. Avoiding complications in abdominal wall surgery. Ann Plast Surg. 2016;76:227–30.
4. Atisha D, Alderman AK. A systematic review of abdominal wall function following abdominal flaps for postmastectomy breast reconstruction. Ann Plast Surg. 2009;63:222–30.
5. Chun YS, Sinha I, Turko A, Yueh JH, Lipsitz S, Pribaz JJ, Lee BT. Comparison of morbidity, functional outcome, and satisfaction following bilateral TRAM versus bilateral DIEP flap breast reconstruction. Plast Reconstr Surg. 2010;126:1133–41.
6. Codner M, Bostwick J, Nahai F, Bried J, Eaves F. TRAM flap vascular delay for high risk breast reconstruction. Plast Reconstr Surg. 1995;96:1615–22.
7. Rozen WM, Ashton MW, Grinsell D. The branching pattern of the deep inferior epigastric artery revisited in-vivo: a new classification based on CT angiography. Clin Anat. 2010;23:87–92.
8. Selber J. Can I make robotic surgery make sense in my practice? Plast Reconstr Surg. 2017;139:781e–92e.
9. daVinciSurgicalSystem.Dockingandtargetingarms.2016.https://us.davincisurgerycommunity. com/detail/videos/p8_or_patient-cart/video/5210231877001/docking-and-targeting-arms?aut oStart=true&index=1.
10. da Vinci Surgical System. Patient clearance button. 2016. https://us.davincisurgerycommunity. com/detail/videos/p3_xi-overview-for-robotic-coordinators/video/5211400171001/ patient-clearance-button?autoStart=true.
11. da Vinci Surgical System. Instrument insertion. 2016. https://us.davincisurgerycommunity. com/detail/videos/p8_or_patient-cart/video/5823026918001/instrument-insertion?autoStart=t rue&index=3.
12. da Vinci Surgical System. Port hopping. 2016. https://us.davincisurgerycommunity.com/detail/ videos/p8_or_patient-cart/video/5211440506001/port-hopping?autoStart=true&index=6.

Selected Reading

Ibrahim A, Sarhane K, Pederson J, Selber J. Robotic harvest of the rectus abdominis muscle: principles and clinical applications. Semin Plast Surg. 2014;28:026–31.
Pedersen J, Song DH, Selber JC. Robotic, intraperitoneal harvest of the rectus abdominis muscle. Plast Reconstr Surg. 2014;134:1057–63.
Selber J. Can I make robotic surgery make sense in my practice? Plast Reconstr Surg. 2017;139:781e–92e.

Robotic Breast Reconstruction with the Latissimus Dorsi Flap

4

Mark W. Clemens and Jesse C. Selber

Introduction

Surgeons have spent the better part of four decades attempting to do more with less, evolving from large open surgical procedures, to laparoscopic approaches, and now finally to robotic-assisted minimally invasive surgery. Robotic-assisted technology has allowed for significant advances in tumor ablation while minimizing surgical morbidity, essentially freeing physicians from the physical limitations of their own hands. Robotic techniques have successfully integrated into urology, surgical oncology, gynecology, and thoracic surgery, but plastic surgical indications remain a relatively novel frontier. For two-stage, delayed-immediate reconstruction of the breast, robotic-assisted latissimus dorsi harvest (RALDH) is an excellent option for patients who wish to avoid a traditional latissimus dorsi donor-site incision (Fig. 4.1). RALDH is associated with a lower complication rates and reliable results for delayed reconstruction of the irradiated breast and eliminates the need for a donor-site incision. In this chapter, we review indications for robotic-assisted surgery in breast reconstruction, pertinent anatomy, patient selection, technique, and institutional outcomes.

Radiation therapy is associated with significant deleterious effects on implant-based breast reconstruction such as malposition, capsular contracture, device extrusion, and therefore the standard of care for reconstruction of the irradiated breast is an autologous tissue [1–3]. Autologous reconstructions should be delayed until after radiation therapy to prevent radiation sequelae such as fat necrosis and tissue fibrosis [4]. Commonly utilized autologous reconstructive options include abdominal-based flaps and the latissimus dorsi muscle flap combined with an implant. Abdominal-based flaps can create a totally autologous reconstruction; however,

M. W. Clemens (✉) · J. C. Selber
Department of Plastic Surgery, MD Anderson Cancer Center, Houston, TX, USA
e-mail: mwclemens@mdanderson.org; jcselber@mdanderson.org

© Springer Nature Switzerland AG 2021
J. C. Selber (ed.), *Robotics in Plastic and Reconstructive Surgery*,
https://doi.org/10.1007/978-3-030-74244-7_4

Fig. 4.1 Delayed-immediate breast reconstruction protocol. (Reprinted with permission from Clemens et al. [14])

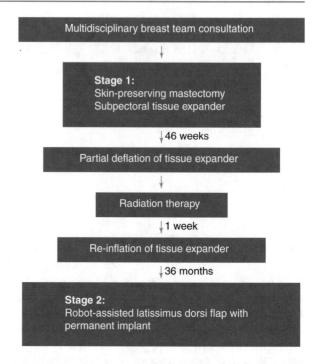

certain patients may not be surgical candidates due to previous abdominal surgeries, failed free flaps, or a paucity of abdominal tissue, and consequently these patients most benefit from a pedicled latissimus dorsi muscle flap breast reconstruction [5].

A two-stage delayed-immediate protocol has been previously described which allows patients that require external beam radiation therapy (EBRT) to receive a skin-preserving mastectomy while avoiding radiation effects associated with an immediate breast reconstruction [6–8]. For the properly selected patient, delayed-immediate breast reconstruction allows for optimal delivery of radiation therapy while still providing patients with the aesthetic benefits of preserving the mastectomy skin envelope and decreasing the adverse effects of radiation therapy.

Robotic-assisted latissimus dorsi harvest (RALDH) has emerged as an integral part of the delayed-immediate protocol at our institution for patients who have successfully completed EBRT with a tissue expander but are not candidates for abdominal-based flaps [9, 10]. The traditional open technique (TOT) of latissimus dorsi harvest can create an obvious donor site scar between 15 and 45 cm in length. Endoscopic latissimus dorsi harvest has been previously shown to result in less subjective patient pain and allowed for earlier and better movement of the upper extremity of the donor site [11, 12]. RALDH utilizes the Da Vinci Robotic Surgical System (Intuitive Surgical Inc., Sunnyvale, CA) to assist in elevation of the latissimus dorsi flap with improved visualization and surgical dexterity over endoscopic harvest and superior cosmetic advantages over the traditional open technique (TOT) by avoiding a back donor-site incision.

Anatomy

RALDH requires familiarity with the pertinent anatomy of the back, axilla, and the latissimus dorsi muscle. The latissimus dorsi muscle is the largest muscle in the upper body and is responsible for extension, adduction, transverse extension also known as horizontal abduction, flexion from an extended position, and (medial) internal rotation of the shoulder joint. The latissimus dorsi muscle derives much of its origin from the thoracolumbar fascia. The latissimus dorsi is innervated by the sixth, seventh, and eighth cervical nerves through the thoracodorsal (long scapular) nerve. The latissimus dorsi muscle has a dual blood supply (Type V) from the subscapular artery and the posterior paraspinous perforators. Both circulatory systems are diffusely interconnected so that the muscle can survive in its entirety if either pedicle is interrupted. The dominant thoracodorsal artery is a branch of the subscapular artery.

With a length of 8.5 cm (range 6.5–12 cm) and approximate diameter of 3 mm (range 2–4 mm). The thoracodorsal artery courses from the axilla along the anterior border of the latissimus dorsi muscle, enters the muscle from underneath, and spreads into two or three major branches at the undersurface of the muscle.

Patient Selection

Patients most benefiting from breast reconstruction with a RALDH have a low BMI, thin body habitus, and athletic where secondary autologous donor sites may be unavailable for reconstruction of the breast. Previous transection of the thoracodorsal artery or vein during a lymphadenectomy is an absolute contraindication and should be taken into account during patient selection. Patients with comorbidities such as smoking, diabetes, and collagen vascular diseases will likely have higher complication rates but are only relative contraindications.

Preoperative Planning and/or Patient Preparation

We perform evaluation of all patients in consultation by a multidisciplinary breast team, which included members of breast oncology, surgical oncology, radiation oncology, and plastic and reconstructive surgery. During surgical stage 1, patients undergo skin-sparing mastectomy and immediate placement of a tissue expander with or without bioprosthetic mesh. Patients are expanded weekly during the 4–6 weeks prior to radiation therapy and then were deflated to 1/3 total fill capacity just prior to initiation of EBRT as per radiation oncology request [13] (Fig. 4.2). Within 1 week of the completion of EBRT, patients are reinflated to original volume. RALDH is performed after 6 months following radiation therapy to allow for soft tissue healing.

The following technical considerations are important for application of RALDH in the delayed-immediate breast reconstruction protocol. Tissue expansion must be

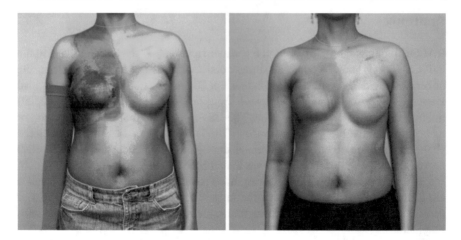

Fig. 4.2 Case example: Delayed-immediate reconstruction of an irradiated breast using a robotic-assisted latissimus dorsi harvest (RALDH). (Reprinted with permission from Clemens et al. [14])

sufficient to allow for the desired volume of final implant and muscle flap, which may require additional expansions after the completion of radiation therapy. If additional volume is required, expansion should be continued at a slower rate, average every 2–3 weeks, until the desired volume is met. For unilateral reconstructions, stage 2 may be combined with a contralateral mastopexy or augmentation for symmetry procedure.

Surgical Technique

Surgery begins with the patient on a bean bag for stabilization in a lateral decubitus positioning. Incision is made through the patient's previous mastectomy skin scar and removal of the tissue expander. Dissection continues into the axilla where the lateral border of the latissimus dorsi muscle is identified. Patency of the thoracodorsal artery and vein is confirmed by Doppler evaluation. Four to six centimeters of dissection is performed on the superficial and deep surface of the latissimus dorsi muscle. Robotic assistance is made utilizing a Da Vinci Robotic System (Intuitive Surgery, Sunnyvale, CA). Robotic harvest technique is performed completely through three access ports/drain sites for robotic instrumentation with no additional incisions required (Fig. 4.3). During muscle transposition, the thoracodorsal nerve is left intact, but the humeral insertion of the muscle is partially divided (80%) to allow for advancement of the muscle and to decrease animation deformity. The pectoralis major muscle that has been providing temporary expander coverage may be fibrosed or constricted from radiation therapy and should not be transected but instead released from the skin envelope and resewn back to the chest wall. Release of the pectoralis muscle from the mastectomy skin flap provides a noncapsular surface for the latissimus flap to adhere. For RALDH opposite a prosthetic

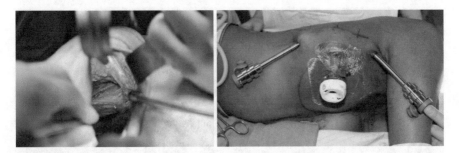

Fig. 4.3 Intraoperative views during RALDH: (Left) Predissection of latissimus dorsi with exposure of thoracodorsal artery and vein. Note all dissection is accomplished through anterior mastectomy incision with no additional skin incisions required. (Right) A 12 and two 8 French ports placed at the lateral border of the latissimus dorsi muscle. (Reprinted with permission from Clemens et al. [14])

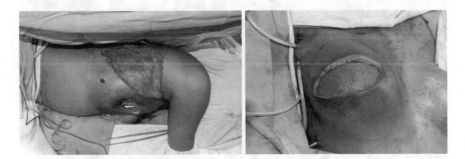

Fig. 4.4 Intraoperative views during RALDH: (Left) Transposition of latissimus dorsi muscle underneath a subcutaneous skin bridge. (Right) Latissimus dorsi muscle achieves total muscle coverage over a permanent silicone-shaped implant (410 FF 425cc, Allergan Corporation, Irvine, CA). Note previous port sites are utilized for drain placement. (Reprinted with permission from Clemens et al. [14])

reconstruction, the same sized implant should be used for both breasts. Despite the addition of the latissimus dorsi, the muscle volume becomes negligible with atrophy and the resolution of swelling. Care should be taken to attempt total latissimus dorsi muscle coverage of the implant from inframammary fold (IMF) to clavicle (Fig. 4.4). Radiation therapy tends to elevate the IMF and required lowering in almost all cases.

Postoperative Care

Postoperative care includes deep venous thrombosis prophylaxis with low molecular weight heparin initiated on postoperative day 1. Hospital course was in general 2–3 days. Routine follow-up included physical examination in an outpatient clinic weekly until drain removal, then at 1 month, and every 3 months for 1 year, and then annually thereafter (Fig. 4.5).

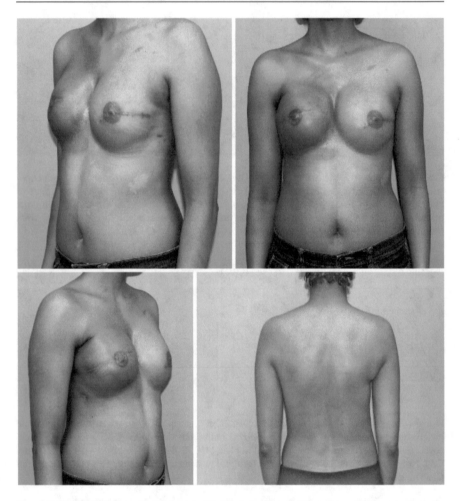

Fig. 4.5 Postoperative results: Patient is 10 months postoperative and has now received nipple construction with areolar tattooing. The patient was noted to have a minor contour defect of her donor site. Her postoperative course was without complication. (Reprinted with permission from Clemens et al. [14])

Clinical Cases and Outcomes

We performed a retrospective review of a consecutive series of 146 pedicled latissimus dorsi muscle flaps performed for breast reconstruction, of which 17 were performed with Da Vinci robotic assistance during the study period (average follow-up 14.6 ± 7.3 months). Latissimus dorsi breast reconstruction following radiation was performed in 76 patients, 64 (84.2%) traditional open technique (TOT) patients (average follow-up 16.4 ± 6.9 months) and 12 (15.8%) RALDH patients (average follow-up 12.3 ± 8.3 months) (Table 4.1). All patients received a stage 1 skin-sparing mastectomy with immediate tissue expander reconstruction. Oncologic

Table 4.1 Patient characteristics and outcomes

Variable	RALDH ($N = 12$)	TOT ($N = 64$)
Average age (years)	54.3	56.1
Previous radiation (%)	100	100
BMI	25.4	25.9
Comorbidities (%)	16.6	18.8
Smokers (%)	25	21.9
Stage 1 bioprosthetic mesh (%)	100	71.2
Surgical complication (%)	16.7	37.5
Seroma	8.3	8.9
Delayed healing	0	7.8
Infection	14.1	8.3
Unplanned reoperation	8.3	12.5
Capsular contracture	0	4.7
Average follow-up (months)	12.3	16.4

Reprinted with permission from Clemens et al. [14]
Abbreviations: *RALDH* robotic-assisted latissimus dorsi harvest, *TOT* traditional open technique, *BMI* body mass index

indications included invasive ductal (85.5%) and invasive lobular carcinoma (14.5%). Patients received an average of 2.8 (range 0–4) expansions initiated between 1 and 2 weeks postoperatively. Radiation therapy was on average 60 Gy with routine inclusion of internal mammary nodes. Stage 2 reconstruction with latissimus dorsi muscle harvest and placement of a permanent implant was performed at an average of 7.1 months (range 3–11 months). All pedicled flaps resulted in successful breast reconstructions. Average time of latissimus dorsi harvest in the TOT technique was 58 minutes (range 42 minutes to 1 hour 38 minutes) compared to RALDH harvest 1 hour 32 minutes (range 1 hour 5 minutes to 2 hours 35 minutes). Average length of hospital stay of the TOT technique was 3.4 days (range 3–6) compared to RALDH harvest 2.7 (range 2–3 days).

Surgical complication rates were statistically equivalent: 37.5% TOT versus 16.7% RALDH ($p = 0.31$) which included seroma (10.9% vs. 8.3%), infection (14.1% vs. 8.3%), wound healing (7.8% vs. 0), and capsular contracture (4.7% vs. 0). No RALDH muscle flaps required converting to an open technique, and all flaps resulted in successful breast reconstructions. Formal muscle strength testing was not performed.

A case example is demonstrated in Fig. 4.2 with a delayed-immediate reconstruction of an irradiated breast using a RALDH. This 42-year-old female was diagnosed with invasive ductal carcinoma od the right breast with positive lymph node metastasis. She was treated with bilateral mastectomies, right axillary dissection, and immediate reconstruction using tissue expanders (133MX 400cc, Allergan Corporation, Irvine, CA) followed by external beam radiation therapy (EBRT, 60 Gy) to the right chest wall. (Left) Immediately and (Right) 6 months following radiation therapy. Note radiation induced constriction and elevation of the right inframammary fold, which must be corrected. At 6 months, she received breast reconstruction with a RALDH over a round silicone implant, and her postoperative course was without any complications or need for revision.

Conclusion

Robotic-assisted surgical techniques have applications in reconstructive surgery of the breast for select patients. The surgical robot is a valuable additional instrument for the reconstructive surgeon's toolkit when approaching challenging cases. Patients most suited for these techniques are two-stage delayed-immediate breast reconstructions in low BMI patients where primary autologous options may be unavailable. Robotic-assisted latissimus dorsi harvest has demonstrated less incisions and scars, faster recovery, improved complication profile, all with modest tradeoffs in cost and operative time. We are confident that plastic surgery indications for the surgical robot will continue to expand, and this technology will become an essential component in the armamentarium of the reconstructive surgeon.

Conflict of Interest None of the authors have any relevant financial relationships or affiliations to disclose.

References

1. Ascherman JA, Hanasono MW, Newman MI, Hughes DB. Implant reconstruction in breast cancer patients with radiation therapy. Plast Reconstr Surg. 2006;117:359–65.
2. Spear SL, Onyewu C. Staged breast reconstruction with saline-filled implants in the irradiated breast: recent trends and therapeutic implications. Plast Reconstr Surg. 2000;105:930–42.
3. Kronowitz SJ, Robb GL. Radiation therapy and breast reconstruction: a critical review of the literature. Plast Reconstr Surg. 2009;124(2):395–408.
4. Tran NV, Chang DW, Gupta A, et al. Comparison of immediate and delayed TRAM flap breast reconstruction in patients receiving postmastectomy radiation therapy. Plast Reconstr Surg. 2001;108:78.
5. Spear SL, Boehmler J, Clemens MW. The latissimus flap in the irradiated breast. In: Spear SL, editor. Surgery of the breast: principles and art. 3rd ed. Philadelphia: Lippincott-Raven; 2011.
6. Kronowitz SJ, Hunt KK, Kuerer HM, et al. Delayed-immediate breast reconstruction. Plast Reconstr Surg. 2004;113:1617.
7. Kronowitz SJ. Immediate versus delayed reconstruction. Clin Plast Surg. 2007;96:39.
8. Kronowitz SJ. Delayed-immediate breast reconstruction: technical and timing considerations. Plast Reconstr Surg. 2010;125(2):463–74.
9. Selber JC. Robotic latissimus dorsi muscle harvest. Plast Reconstr Surg. 2011;128:88e–90e.
10. Selber JC, Baumann DP, Holsinger FC. Robotic latissimus dorsi muscle harvest: a case series. Plast Reconstr Surg. 2012;129(6):1305–12.
11. Lin CH, Wei FC, Levin LS, Chen MC. Donor-site morbidity comparison between endoscopically assisted and traditional harvest of free latissimus dorsi muscle flap. Plast Reconstr Surg. 1999;104:1070–7; quiz 1078; review erratum Plast Reconstr Surg. 2000;105:823.
12. Pomel C, Missana MC, Lasser P. Endoscopic harvesting of the latissimus dorsi flap in breast reconstructive surgery: feasibility study and review of the literature. Ann Chir. 2002;127:337–42.
13. Motwami SB, Strom EA, Schechter NR, et al. The impact of immediate breast reconstruction on the technical delivery of postmastectomy radiotherapy. Int J Radiat Oncol Biol Phys. 2006;66:76.
14. Clemens MW, Kronowitz S, Selber JC. Robotic-assisted latissimus dorsi harvest in delayed-immediate breast reconstruction. Semin Plast Surg. 2014;28(1):20–5.

The RoboDIEP: Robotic-Assisted Deep Inferior Epigastric Perforator Flaps for Breast Reconstruction

5

Sarah N. Bishop and Jesse C. Selber

Introduction

The ideal breast reconstruction maximizes recipient site specificity by supplying "like with like," and minimizes donor site morbidity. The goal of the deep inferior epigastric perforator (DIEP) flap is to achieve this ideal. Although the majority of breast reconstruction in the United States is implant-based reconstruction, studies have shown that patients are most satisfied long term with autologous reconstruction [1–8]. There has been a significant evolution to decrease the morbidity of abdominal wall dissection in autologous breast reconstruction. The pedicled transverse rectus abdominis myocutaneous (TRAM) flap preceded the DIEP in breast reconstruction [9]. The pedicled TRAM not only sacrifices all of the rectus muscle, but it is perfused by the less dominant superior epigastric vessels and can lead to ischemia, congestion, and fat necrosis of the flap. The delay principle allowed for the pedicled TRAM to improve its survivability off the less dominant superior epigastric system; however, this predisposes the patient to an additional surgery [10]. The free TRAM allowed the flap to be perfused by the dominant inferior epigastric system and enabled improved mobility for inset [11]. However, both the pedicled and free TRAM flap completely sacrifice the rectus muscles, leading to significant weakness of the anterior abdominal wall and a high risk of bulge and hernia formation. The muscle-sparing TRAM (ms-TRAM) was the first effort to decrease abdominal wall morbidity and a classification scheme was developed to describe what part of the muscle is removed [12]. The DIEP was first described in 1989 by Koshima and Soeda and was ultimately popularized by Allen and Blondeel [13–15], and has the advantage of removing no muscle. The amount of muscle spared has been shown in some studies to correlate with a decrease in abdominal wall morbidity [16]. The DIEP was further refined by not only preserving the

S. N. Bishop · J. C. Selber (✉)
Department of Plastic Surgery, MD Anderson Cancer Center, Houston, TX, USA
e-mail: Bishops@ccf.org; jcselber@mdanderson.org

© Springer Nature Switzerland AG 2021
J. C. Selber (ed.), *Robotics in Plastic and Reconstructive Surgery*,
https://doi.org/10.1007/978-3-030-74244-7_5

muscle but also by preserving the segmental nerves of the rectus muscle [17]. Muscle bulging can occur after muscle-sparing surgery if the muscle is denervated. Over time, more and more attention has been placed on the importance of protecting the native anatomy to restore preoperative function. Yet even in removing no muscle, a significant amount of muscle damage is done during the traditional open DIEP simply by dissecting the perforator and pedicle through the muscle and fascia. To date, there has been no way to avoid this seemingly necessary evil in harvesting the DIEP, and bulging below the arcuate line is a common long term side effect. This causes significant discomfort to women who undergo autologous breast reconstruction.

The next step in improving the donor site morbidity from the DIEP flap harvest is to limit the anterior muscular and fascial dissection. Traditionally, the DIEP flap is harvested in its entirety from an anterior open approach. Because most of the pedicle lies deep to the rectus muscle leading into the pelvis, a large fascial incision is usually required even if one only perforator is selected. Morbidity from the fascial incision is increased because a substantial portion of this incision is below the arcuate line (Fig. 5.1), where the anterior abdominal wall contributes most of the structural integrity. Furthermore, the muscle frequently needs to be split or lifted laterally to facilitate harvesting the flap as the main pedicle runs along the under surface of the rectus muscle. Splitting the muscle damages the muscle and can also lead to damaging segmental neurovascular bundles that supply the rectus from lateral to medial, predisposing the patient to muscular bulging from de-functionalized muscle. However, if a posterior approach is used to dissect the pedicle, the anterior anatomy is preserved in situ and the fascial incision can be limited. Limiting the fascial incision and retaining the native neurovasculature should have a great impact on reducing hernia, bulging, and abdominal discomfort. By further minimizing the morbidity of the donor site of DIEP flaps, the goal of perforator flaps is truly achieved: do as little harm as possible.

Fig. 5.1 Bilateral DIEP: left side (page right) open technique, right side (page left) RoboDIEP technique. This demonstrates both favorable versus unfavorable anatomy for a RoboDIEP, and also the amount of abdominal morbidity that can be spared with favorable anatomy and a robotic approach

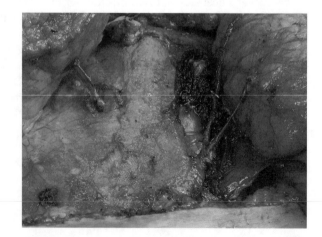

The first robotic surgery was the Programmable Universal Machine for Assembly 200 (PUMA) used in a neurosurgical case on a human patient to obtain a precise and delicate biopsy in 1985 [18, 19]. The success of this endeavor led to the use of robots in urologic surgery with the Surgeon-Assisted Robot for Prostatectomy (SARP), Prostate Robot (PROBOT), and the UROBOT [18, 20]. However, these robots functioned by the use of fixed anatomical landmarks and were not translatable to other surgeries requiring dynamic ability [18]. This ultimately led to the development of the da Vinci® robot which is today the most widely used robotic system worldwide [21]. The da Vinci® works as an "operator-effector," or "command-control" device whereby the surgeon works at a console using remote manipulators to control the patient-facing robotic system.

Use of the robot overcomes many of the challenges of laparoscopic surgery to become the next frontier in minimally invasive surgery. Robotic surgery offers 3D magnified vision, physiologic tremor filtering, motion scaling, and instruments capable of seven degrees of freedom, as well as ergonomic surgeon positioning. It is widely accepted that the robot offers superior advantage in small spaces such as the pelvis and has led to the dominance of robotic surgery in urologic and gynecologic surgery [22, 23]. Because of its precision and minimally invasive capabilities, use of the robot has since been extrapolated to all types of general surgery, head and neck surgery, gynecology oncology surgery, plastic surgery and is even being considered for its potential in microsurgical applications [24]. In performing the RoboDIEP, the surgeon capitalizes on both the technical superiority of the robotic system, combined with the minimally invasive benefits of the posterior approach that promises to limit abdominal wall morbidity.

Patient Selection

The use of computed tomography angiography (CTA) in preoperative planning has been shown to decrease operative time and improve outcomes [25, 26]. Preoperative imaging in RoboDIEPs is essential in determining candidacy for the robotic approach. A patient with a single or two closely grouped perforators with a short intramuscular course will benefit most from a robotic DIEP. If a larger number of perforators are used or required, then more anterior/open dissection is required, thus decreasing the advantage of the posterior robotic approach.

A rough mathematical equation, $B = C - A$, can be used to quantify the potential benefit (B) of using the robotic approach. Here B is defined as the *Benefit*, or the reduction in the length of the fascial incision, A is the length of the *intramuscular course* (determined from the CT scan), and C is the entire *length of the pedicle* (from the perforator to the origin at the external iliacs). For instance, if the pedicle length, C, is 13.5 cm (this is typical), the intramuscular course, A, is 3 cm, then Benefit, B, or length of fascial incision spared is roughly 10.5 cm, a significant savings! This calculation appears to be reliable and can be presented to the patient preoperatively and corroborated intra-operatively with photo-documentation.

Technique

The Robotic DIEP commences with the elevation of the abdominal flaps as in the traditional open version. The preselected perforator is identified and a small fascial incision is made around the perforator and dissected to only where the perforator exits the deep surface of the rectus muscle (Fig. 5.2). Unlike the open version where the fascial incision is extended for access to the pedicle, in the RoboDIEP the open dissection stops just at the perforator level. At this point, pneumoperitoneum is established and insufflation is set to between 10 and 15 mmHg. In our practice, we use a Veress needle followed by an AirSeal port (CONMED, Utica NY). Three robotic 8 mm ports are then placed directly through the fascia along a line connecting the anterior axillary line and the anterior superior iliac spine (ASIS). All three ports are placed on the contralateral side of the flap being harvested. The most cephalad port is close to the costal margin, and the most caudal port is close to the ASIS (Fig. 5.3). Port placement is as lateral to the semilunar line of the rectus muscle as possible in order to optimize the angle of approach to the deep inferior epigastric pedicle. The remaining third port is placed equidistant between the cephalad and caudal port and is used as the camera port. Since the ports are placed directly through the fascia, there is no skin and fat to traverse. In addition, ports are placed directly under vision using a 5mm laparoscopic camera through the insufflation port, making placement very safe and reliable.

The da Vinci® surgical robot (Intuitive Surgical, Sunnyvale CA) is positioned at the bedside on the ipsilateral side of the flap at 90°. The arms are docked in the usual fashion. The operating surgeon is now at the console, and monopolar scissors and bipolar graspers are placed in the cephalad and caudal ports. The course of the inferior epigastric vessels along the under surface of the rectus is identified just beneath the thin peritoneal lining. The peritoneum is opened sharply and the deep inferior epigastric pedicle is dissected to its origin at the external iliacs. The dissection is continued cephalad to dissect the pedicle off of the rectus muscle and traced up into

Fig. 5.2 RoboDIEP fascial incision is only necessary around the perforator/s

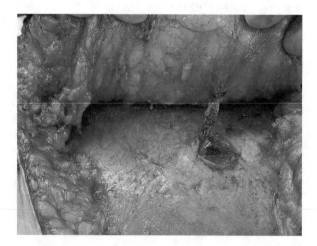

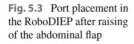

Fig. 5.3 Port placement in the RoboDIEP after raising of the abdominal flap

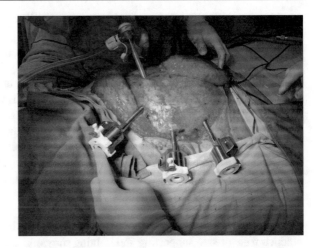

the fascial defect, connecting it to the aperture in the fascia that was made from above during the open perforator dissection. Some gas will leak as the fascial opening is approached, and this can be controlled by gentle pressure with a moist lap pad.

After the pedicle is dissected complete, the pedicle is then clipped, divided, and extracted through the fascial defect. A barbed suture is then passed through a port, and the posterior sheath is closed robotically with a running suture. The tension on the posterior rectus sheath closure can be minimized by decreasing the pneumoperitoneum to 8 mmHg. Either the da Vinci® Si or Xi systems are appropriate for this surgery; however, the Xi has arms on a boom that can rotate around the patient without moving the base. This feature is helpful in bilateral reconstructions where a separate docking procedure is required for each side. After the flap is removed, the ports are removed and fascial incisions closed externally with "figure of 8" sutures. The remainder of the case proceeds as a routine DIEP.

In our early experience, we have limited the fascial incision to an average of 2–3 cm. This technique has reduced postoperative pain and length of stay and enhanced overall recovery. We anticipate that the significantly decreased fascial incision and muscular dissection will also lead to decreased hernia and bulg rates, although long-term data and comparisons to traditional DIEP flaps will be needed to definitely demonstrate this long-term benefit.

Discussion

The DIEP represents a significant improvement over the free TRAM by decreasing abdominal morbidity and pain and increasing long-term core strength and function. However, DIEP flaps performed in the traditional open fashion still have a large fascial incision and muscle splitting and dissection that can still lead to hernia and bulging. Hernia after DIEP has been quoted to range from 0% to 7% and bulging from 2.3% to 33% depending on the series [27–32]. By decreasing the fascial incision and muscle splitting and avoiding neurovascular damage to the muscle, one would expect a significant decrease in pain, an expedited recovery, and decreases in hernias and bulge rates.

As with any new skill acquisition, there is a learning curve associated with robotic surgery in general and the RoboDIEP specifically. Prior to commencing this technique, one should go through proper observation and training on the robot. Working with experienced urology or colorectal surgeons who are comfortable with port placement and the robotic system is helpful for the first handful of cases. As with any intra-abdominal operation, inadvertent injury to viscera is possible, although we have not encountered it. A full-service hospital setting is recommended in case of the need for general surgery assistance. A team-based approach is also critical for patient safety and includes the console surgeon, patient-side assistant, anesthesiologist, scrub technician, and circulator who are all familiar with robotic surgery [33].

Intuitive offers online modules accompanied by simulation and a lab-based practicum devoted to supporting and training surgeons. These simulations should be completed by anyone serious about embarking on this technique [34]. Hospital credentialing typically requires being proctored by someone (usually a urologist) experienced in robotic surgery for a specified number of cases that will be specific to the bylaws of the hospital set forth by the medical staff and/or medical practice committee [33, 35].

Conclusion

The RoboDIEP offers women a less invasive approach to DIEP flap reconstructions. The morbidity of hernia, muscle bulge forrmation, and potential loss of core strength should be minimized by decreasing the fascial and muscular damage incurred during traditional open surgery. The ideal patient characteristics are those with single or closely grouped perforators with a short intramuscular course. In patients who are good anatomic candidates, the benefit from the robotic DIEP is substantial.

References

1. Damen TH, Mureau MA, Timman R, et al. The pleasing end result after DIEP flap breast reconstruction: a review of additional operations. J Plast Reconstr Aesthet Surg. 2009;62:71–6.
2. Tønseth KA, Hokland BM, Tindholdt TT, et al. Patient-reported outcomes after breast reconstruction with deep inferior epigastric perforator flaps. Scand J Plast Reconstr Surg Hand Surg. 2007;41:173–7.
3. Tønseth KA, Hokland BM, Tindholdt TT, et al. Quality of life, patient satisfaction and cosmetic outcome after breast reconstruction using DIEP flap or expandable breast implant. J Plast Reconstr Aesthet Surg. 2008;61:1188–94.
4. Yueh JH, Slavin SA, Adesiyun T, et al. Patient satisfaction in postmastectomy breast reconstruction: a comparative evaluation of DIEP, TRAM, latissimus flap, and implant techniques. Plast Reconstr Surg. 2010;125:1585–95.
5. Damen TH, Timman R, Kunst EH, et al. High satisfaction rates in women after DIEP flap breast reconstruction. J Plast Reconstr Aesthet Surg. 2010;63:93–100.

6. Damen TH, Wei W, Mureau MA, et al. Medium-term cost analysis of breast reconstructions in a single Dutch centre: a comparison of implants, implants preceded by tissue expansion, LD transpositions and DIEP flaps. J Plast Reconstr Aesthet Surg. 2011;64:1043–53.
7. Liu C, Zhuang Y, Momeni A, et al. Quality of life and patient satisfaction after microsurgical abdominal flap versus staged expander/implant breast reconstruction: a critical study of unilateral immediate breast reconstruction using patient-reported outcomes instrument BREAST-Q. Breast Cancer Res Treat. 2014;146:117–26.
8. Thorarinsson A, Fröjd V, Kölby L, Ljungal J, Taft C, Mark H. Long-term health-related quality of life after breast reconstruction: comparing 4 different methods of reconstruction. Plast Reconstr Surg Glob Open. 2017;5(6):e1316.
9. Hartrampf CR, Scheflan M, Black PW. Breast reconstruction with a transverse abdominal island flap. Plast Reconstr Surg. 1982;69(2):216–25.
10. Moon HK, Taylor GI. The vascular anatomy of rectus abdominis musculocutaneous flaps based on the deep superior epigastric system. Plast Reconstr Surg. 1988;82:815–32. 23.
11. Grotting JC. The free abdominoplasty flap for immediate breast reconstruction. Ann Plast Surg. 1991;27(4):351–4.
12. Nahabedian MY, Momen B, Galdino G, Manson PN. Breast reconstruction with the free TRAM or DIEP flap: patient selection, choice of flap, and outcome. Plast Reconstr Surg. 2002;110:466–75; discussion 476–7.
13. Koshima I, Soeda S. Inferior epigastric artery skin flaps without rectus abdominis muscle. Br J Plast Surg. 1989;42:645–8.
14. Allen RJ, Treece P. Deep inferior epigastric perforator flap for breast reconstruction. Ann Plast Surg. 1994;32:32.
15. Blondeel PN. One hundred DIEP flap breast reconstructions: a personal experience. Br J Plast Surg. 1999;52:104.
16. Selber JC, et al. A prospective study comparing the functional impact of SIEA, DIEP, and muscle-sparing free TRAM flaps on the abdominal wall: Part II. Bilateral reconstruction. Plast Reconstr Surg. 2010;126(5):1438–53.
17. Lee BT, Chen C, Nguyen MD, Lin SJ, Tobias AM. A new classification system for muscle and nerve preservation in DIEP flap breast reconstruction. Microsurgery. 2010;30:85–90.
18. Abdul-Muhsin H, Patel V. History of robotic surgery. In: Kim CH, editor. Robotics in general surgery. New York: Springer; 2014. p. 3–8.
19. Kwoh YS, Hou J, Jonckheere EA, et al. A robot with improved absolute positioning accuracy for CT guided stereotactic brain surgery. IEEE Trans Biomed Eng. 1988;35(2):153–60.
20. Davies BL, Hibber RD, Ng WS, et al. The development of a surgeon robot for prostatectomies. Proc Inst Mech Eng H. 1991;205:35–8. 12.
21. Leal Ghezzi T, Campos Corleta O. 30 years of robotic surgery. World J Surg. 2016;40:2550–7.
22. Hagen ME, Stein H, Curet MJ. Introduction to the robotic system. In: Kim CH, editor. Robotics in general surgery. New York: Springer; 2014. p. 9–16. 22.
23. Taffinder N, Smith SGT, Huber J, et al. The effect of a second-generation 3D endoscope on the laparoscopic precision of novices and experienced surgeons. Surg Endosc. 1999;13:1087–92. 23.
24. Van Mulken TJM, Boymans CAEM, Schols RM, Cau R, Schoenmakers FBF, Hoekstra LT, Qiu SS, Selber JC, van der Hulst RRWJ. Preclinical experience using a new robotic system created for microsurgery. Plast Reconstr Surg. 2018;142(5):1367–76.
25. Lee KT, Mun GH. Perfusion of the DIEP flaps: a systematic review with meta-analysis. Microsurgery. 2018;38(1):98e108.
26. O'Connor EF, Rozen WM, Chowdhry M, Band B, Ramakrishnan VV, Griffiths M. Preoperative computed tomography angiography for planning DIEP flap breast reconstruction reduces operative time and overall complications. Gland Surg. 2016;5(2):93e8.
27. Futter CM, Webster MH, Hagen S, et al. A retrospective comparison of abdominal muscle strength following breast reconstruction with a free TRAM or DIEP flap. Br J Plast Surg. 2000;53:578–83.

28. Shubinets V, Fox JP, Sarik JR, et al. Surgically treated hernia following abdominally based autologous breast reconstruction: prevalence, outcomes, and expenditures. Plast Reconstr Surg. 2016;137:749–57.
29. Mennie JC, Mohanna PN, O'Donoghue JM, et al. Donor-site hernia repair in abdominal flap breast reconstruction: a population-based cohort study of 7929 patients. Plast Reconstr Surg. 2015;136:1–9.
30. Tomouk T, Mohan AT, Azizi A, et al. Donor site morbidity in DIEP free flap breast reconstructions: a comparison of unilateral, bilateral, and bipedicled surgical procedure types. J Plast Reconstr Aesthet Surg. 2017;70:1505–13.
31. Ingvaldsen CA, Bosse G, Mynarek GK, et al. Donor-site morbidity after DIEAP flap breast reconstruction-a 2-year postoperative computed tomography comparison. Plast Reconstr Surg Glob Open. 2017;5:e1405.
32. Uda H, Kamochi H, Sarukawa S, et al. Clinical and quantitative isokinetic comparison of abdominal morbidity and dynamics following DIEP versus muscle-sparing free TRAM flap breast reconstruction. Plast Reconstr Surg. 2017;140:1101–9.
33. Ben-Or S, Nifong LW, Chitwood WR Jr. Robotic surgical training. Cancer J. 2013;19(2):120–3.
34. da Vinci Surgery Online Community Training Program: da Vinci Surgery Clinical Pathway Surgeons.
35. Lenihan JP. Navigating, credentialing, privileging, and learning curves in robotics with an evidence and experienced-based approach. Clin Obstet Gynecol. 2011;54:382–90.

Robotic Nerve and Upper Extremity Surgery

6

Nicola Santelmo, Fred Xavier, and Philippe Liverneaux

Introduction

Microsurgery was developed in the 1960s from experimental work in animals. The first vascular microsurgical anastomosis was performed in a rat in 1960 [1] and the first ear replantation in a rabbit in 1966 [2]. Very quickly, applications were described in humans, and the first replantation of the thumb was published in 1965 [3]. Numerous applications have subsequently been described in human clinical practice, including vascular microsurgery and peripheral nerve microsurgery. As regard to vascular microsurgery, technical advances have made it possible to successively perform replantations, free flaps, pedicled flaps and, more recently, perforator flaps [4]. Regarding microsurgery of the peripheral nerves, technical advances have made it possible to successively perform nerve sutures and nerve grafts, brachial plexus reconstructions, nerve transfers, and recently terminolateral nerve sutures [5].

Since the 1960s, microsurgery has undergone considerable development in its surgical indications, but no major technical advances have been observed, either visually or instrumentally. Although the operating microscopes are now digital, their magnification has not changed. These are always exoscopes that cannot penetrate inside the body. The instruments are now made of titanium, but their handling has not changed. They are always bulky instruments that cannot penetrate inside the body. A technological leap is observed in all industrial fields every 50 years. It is a

N. Santelmo
Department of Thoracic Surgery, University Hospital of Strasbourg, Strasbourg, France
e-mail: nicolas.santelmo@chru-strasbourg.fr

F. Xavier
Orthopedic Surgery, Biomedical Engineering, Cincinnati, OH, USA

P. Liverneaux (✉)
Department of Hand Surgery, SOS Main, CCOM, University Hospital of Strasbourg, FMTS, University of Strasbourg, Strasbourg, France
e-mail: Philippe.liverneaux@chru-strasbourg.fr

© Springer Nature Switzerland AG 2021
J. C. Selber (ed.), *Robotics in Plastic and Reconstructive Surgery*,
https://doi.org/10.1007/978-3-030-74244-7_6

safe bet that robotics will be the technological leap of microsurgery for two main reasons, optical and instrumental. Robotics allows the use of endoscopes that can penetrate inside the body through minimally invasive routes. Robotics further allows the use of miniaturized instruments to subtract the physiological tremor and reduce the movements by the microsurgeon.

Robot-assisted microsurgery or telemicrosurgery offers two major advantages over conventional microsurgery: the minimally invasive surgical approaches and the use of more ergonomic hand gestures by reducing the movements.

Robot-assisted microsurgery is of interest in the two major applications of microsurgery, vascular microsurgery [6] and peripheral nerve microsurgery [7]. Although many prototypes have been recently designed, the Da Vinci® robot is currently the only one used in clinical practice [8]. Microsurgery-specific instruments have been developed, such as the Black Diamond® clamps and the Pott® scissors, as well as microsurgical imaging devices such as a micro-Doppler for detecting inframillimetric vessels [9]. Using these instruments and devices requires a learning curve [10]. The learning of robot-assisted microsurgery follows rules identical to those of conventional microsurgery and specific rules [11], validated by precise evaluation methods [12, 13].

Regarding nerve microsurgery of peripheral nerves, many experimental techniques have been described. The feasibility of microsurgical nerve anastomoses has been demonstrated in the rat sciatic nerve [7] and numerous nerve transfers in brachial plexus palsies such as intercostal nerve [14], phrenic nerve [15], the contralateral transfer of the C7 root of the brachial plexus by two approaches [16] and a minimally invasive technique [17], the description of new approaches for the lower brachial plexus [18], the axillary nerve, and the nerve of the long head triceps [19] in the human anatomical subject.

The main clinical applications of robot-assisted peripheral nerve microsurgery are direct brachial plexus repairs by root [20] and indirect nerve transfusions of the long triceps nerve on the axillary nerve [21, 22], and of a motor fascicle of the ulnar nerve on the motor branch of the musculocutaneous nerve [23]. Some neurolyses have been proposed, such as the lateral femoral cutaneous nerve in the course of a meralgia paresthetica [24] or the median nerve in the carpal tunnel [25], as well as resection of nerve tumors [26, 27].

Clinical Case

A clinical case of robot-assisted transfer of intercostal nerves to the motor branch of the musculocutaneous nerve for the biceps muscle via intrathoracic minimally invasive approach is presented here.

The robot-assisted microsurgery described herein by way of example relates to the peripheral nerves. The aim of this procedure is to recover the most important function in the event of complete paralysis of the brachial plexus: active flexion of the elbow. This is the robot-assisted transfer of intercostal nerves to the motor branch of the musculocutaneous nerve for the biceps muscle by intrathoracic minimally invasive approaches. The conventional technique for harvesting intercostal nerves requires a very extensive incision of dozens of centimeters [28]. The advantage of robot-assisted microsurgical techniques is to use only four incisions of 1 cm each for the placement of the tubes and the exit of the intercostal nerves from the thorax.

There is no specific planning for robotics in this indication. A trained thoracic surgeon must do the trocar placement. A history of major thoracic trauma that could have caused intercostal nerve damage on the side to be operated is a relative contraindication.

The procedure is performed in two stages, the first in lateral decubitus to harvest the intercostal nerves, and the second in supine position to carry out the nerve transfer.

At the first stage, the patient is placed in lateral decubitus, on the opposite side to the surgical site. General anesthesia is performed with contralateral unipulmonary ventilation by selective intubation using a Carlens probe to clear the intrathoracic workspace. The incisions for the tubes are drawn against the eighth intercostal space so that all the instruments and endoscope can converge on the third and fourth intercostal spaces (Fig. 6.1). The endoscopic camera trocar is installed first. A Da Vinci SI® [Intuitive Surgical ™, Sunnyvale, CA, USA] robot is placed at the patient's

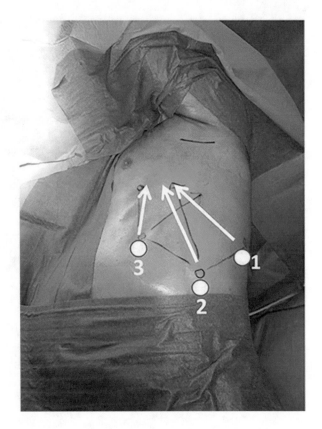

Fig. 6.1 Preparation of surgical approaches. The patient is placed in the left lateral decubitus. Three incisions of 1 cm each are drawn along the eighth intercostal space in front of the axillary line [1], opposite the axillary line [2], and behind the axillary line [3]. Incisions 1 and 3 are designed to accommodate the instrumental tubes, and incision 2, the camera trocar of the Da Vinci® robot. The tubes must allow the instruments and the camera to stay in the workspace, along the third and fourth intercostal spaces

head, and its arms are deployed in such a way that the amplitude of movement of the instruments and of the endoscopic camera allows access to the full length of the intercostal nerves to be taken, that is to say from the mammary artery, in the front, to the pleural dome, in the rear (Fig. 6.2). An insufflation of approximately 12 mmHg is done on the endoscopic camera trocar to enlarge the workspace and reduce the parietal bleeding. During the nerve harvesting phase, a bipolar Maryland® forceps and a pair of curved scissors are used.

In the first stage, the dissection begins with the most cranial intercostal nerve, in order to prevent the bleeding of the caudal nerve from flowing over the most cranial nerve and interfere with its dissection. In the present case, the dissection of the intercostal nerve of the fourth space will begin before that of the third space. The parietal pleura is then carefully opened at the lower edge of the rib to identify the nerve to be harvested without any damage (Fig. 6.3). As soon as the nerve is located, the parietal pleura is incised all along the nerve path, from the mammary artery to the pleural dome. The nerve is then freed from all its attachments along its length and its sensory branches are severed. When the intercostal nerves and third and fourth spaces are completely released, the anterior extremities of the two nerves are cut near their anterior end (Fig. 6.4). A trocar is inserted between the two nerves at their posterior ends in the axilla to recover their anterior ends and to make them

Fig. 6.2 Installation of the Da Vinci® robot. The patient is placed in the left lateral decubitus. The Da Vinci® robot is placed at the patient's head

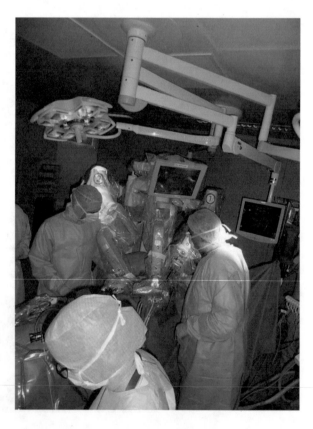

Fig. 6.3 Intrathoracic view. Beginning of dissection of the nerve of the fourth intercostal space [arrow]. The instruments cut the parietal pleura along the fourth intercostal space to reveal the nerve

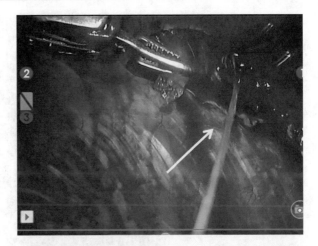

Fig. 6.4 Intrathoracic view. End of the dissection of the nerves of the third and fourth intercostal spaces [arrows]. The nerves have been severed at their anterior extremity and remain. The instruments look for the point of entry of the trocar intended to remove the intercostal nerves from their posterior extremities

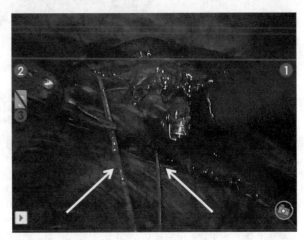

leave the thorax with the aid of an atraumatic forceps. The two intercostal nerves are then exposed on the skin, wrapped in a moist compress, all applied hermetically by an adhesive dressing to avoid damage during the patient's position change (Fig. 6.5). A thoracic drain is placed before modifying the lateral decubitus to supine position.

In the second stage, the patient is placed in supine position and the upper limb to operate rests on a surgical arm table. The incision is drawn on the medial side of the arm to give access to the motor branch of the musculocutaneous nerve for the biceps muscle. The Da Vinci® robot is placed at the side edge of the patient's arm, and the arms of the robot are deployed so that the instruments work on the medial edge of the patient's arm. During the microsurgical suture phase of the intercostal nerves with the motor branch of the musculocutaneous nerve, two Black Diamond® clamps and a pair of Pott® scissors are used.

In the second stage, after change of position, dissection begins with the musculocutaneous nerve whose motor branch for the biceps muscle is individualized as

Fig. 6.5 Extrathoracic
view. The nerves of the
third and fourth intercostal
spaces have been removed
from the thorax by their
anterior extremity [arrows]

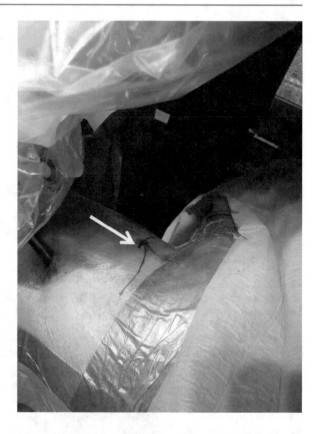

near as possible and then cut into the axilla to obtain a maximum length. A subcutaneous tunnel is made using a long clamp to connect the incision from the thorax of the intercostal nerves to the incision of the arm to the axilla. The nerve ends on the one hand of the motor branch of the musculocutaneous nerve for the biceps muscle and on the other hand of the two intercostal nerves are confronted and then sutured using the robot Da Vinci SI® with 2 points of nylon 10/0 (Fig. 6.6). Biological glue is applied all around the suture area. The incisions are closed in a cutaneous plane without drainage.

In postoperative care, the operated upper limb is immobilized in a vest elbow to the body to avoid stressing the nerve suture and failure. The thoracic drain is removed on the second day, and the patient can return home on the third day. The patient is seen again in the third week to remove the elbow to the body, the dressing, and the sutures. The rehabilitation of maintenance of joint mobility is undertaken for 6 weeks, and the patient is reviewed at the sixth month postoperative, to watch for the first signs of nerve recovery. The active flexion of the elbow is generally obtained at the end of the first year (Figs. 6.7 and 6.8).

Fig. 6.6 Axillary view. The incision out of the thorax nerves of the third and fourth intercostal spaces was closed [yellow arrow]. Result of the robot-assisted microsurgical suture of the two intercostal nerves [black arrow] with the motor branch of the biceps nerve [white arrow]

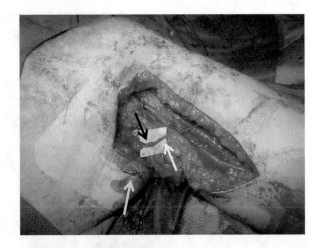

Fig. 6.7 Result after 1 year. The scars are hardly visible

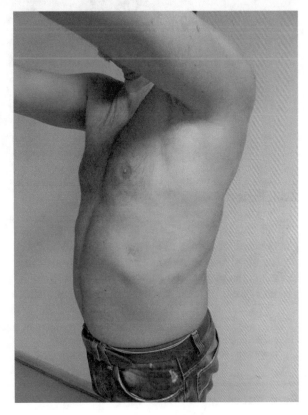

Fig. 6.8 Result after
1 year. The flexion of the
elbow is recovered

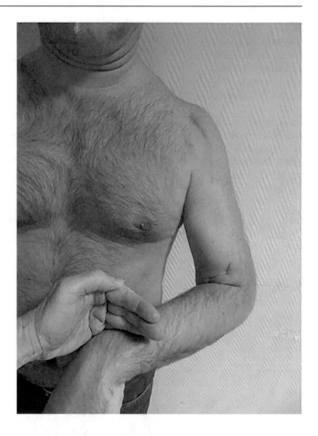

Conclusion

The advantage of robotics in microsurgery is the increase in ergonomics for the
surgeon and the reduction of scars for the patient.

The disadvantage of robotics in microsurgery are the absence of a dedicated
device on the market, the abandonment of the motion reduction in the most recent
versions of the Da Vinci® robots, and a lack of microsurgical Instrumentation.

Conflicts of Interest Philippe Liverneaux has conflicts of interest with Newclip Technics,
Argomedical, Caresyntax.

None of the other authors have conflicts of interest.

References

1. Jacobson JH, Suarez EL. Microsurgery in anastomosis of small vessels. Surg Forum.
   1960;11:243–5.
2. Buncke HJ, Schulz WP. Total ear reimplantation in the rabbit utilizing microminiature vascular
   anastomosis. Br J Plast Surg. 1966;19:15–22.

3. Komatsu S, Tamai S. Successful replantation of a completely cut-off thumb. Plast Reconstr Surg. 1968;42:374–7.
4. Koshima I, Soeda S. Inferior epigastric skin flaps without rectus abdominis muscle. Br J Plast Surg. 1989;42:645–8.
5. Viterbo F, Trindade JC, Hoshino K, Mazzoni NA. End-to-side neurorrhaphy with removal of the epineurial sheath: an experimental study in rats. Plast Reconstr Surg. 1994;94:1038–47.
6. Saleh DB, Syed M, Kulendren D, Ramakrishnan V, Liverneaux PA. Plastic and reconstructive robotic microsurgery--a review of current practices. Ann Chir Plast Esthet. 2015;60:305–12.
7. Nectoux E, Taleb C, Liverneaux P. Nerve repair in telemicrosurgery: an experimental study. J Reconstr Microsurg. 2009;25:261–5.
8. Mattos LS, Caldwell DG, Peretti G, Mora F, Guastini L, Cingolani R. Microsurgery robots: addressing the needs of high-precision surgical interventions. Swiss Med Wkly. 2016;26:1–14.
9. Brahmbhatt JV, Gudeloglu A, Liverneaux P, Parekattil SJ. Robotic microsurgery optimization. Arch Plast Surg. 2014;41:225–30.
10. Ramdhian RM, Bednar M, Mantovani GR, Facca SA, Liverneaux PA. Microsurgery and Telemicrosurgery training: a comparative study. J Reconstr Microsurg. 2011;279:537–42.
11. Liverneaux PA, Hendriks S, Selber JC, Parekattil SJ. Robotically assisted microsurgery: development of basic skills course. Arch Plast Surg. 2013;40:320–6.
12. Alrasheed T, Liu J, Hanasono MM, Butler CE, Selber JC. Robotic microsurgery: validating an assessment tool and plotting the learning curve. Plast Reconstruct Surg. 2014;134:794–803.
13. Alrasheed T, Selber JC. Robotic microsurgical training and evaluation. Semin Plast Surg. 2014;28:5–10.
14. Miyamoto H, Serradori T, Mikami Y, Selber J, Santelmo N, Facca S, Liverneaux P. Robotic intercostal nerve harvest: a feasibility study in a pig model. J Neurosurg. 2016;1241:264–8.
15. Porto De Melo P, Miyamoto H, Serradori T, Ruggiero Mantovani G, Selber J, Facca S, Xu WD, Santelmo N, Liverneaux P. Robotic phrenic nerve harvest: a feasibility study in a pig model. Chir Main. 2014;335:356–60.
16. Jiang S, Ichihara S, Prunières G, Peterson B, Facca S, Xu WD, Liverneaux P. Robot-assisted C7 nerve root transfer from the contralateral healthy side: a preliminary cadaver study. Hand Surg Rehabil. 2016;352:95–9.
17. Bijon C, Chih-Sheng L, Chevallier D, Tran N, Xavier F, Liverneaux P. Endoscopic robot-assisted C7 nerve root retrophalangeal transfer from the contralateral healthy side: a cadaver feasibility study. Ann Chir Plast Esthet. 2017;pii: S0294-1260(17)30073-0. https://doi.org/10.1016/j.anplas.2017.05.004. [Epub ahead of print]
18. Tetik C, Uzun M. Novel axillary approach for brachial plexus in robotic surgery: a cadaveric experiment. Minim Invasive Surg. 2014;2014:927456.
19. Porto De Melo PM, Garcia JC, Montero EF, Atik T, Robert EG, Facca S, Liverneaux PA. Feasibility of an endoscopic approach to the axillary nerve and the nerve to the long head of the triceps Brachii with the help of the Da Vinci robot. Chir Main. 2013;324:206–9.
20. Garcia JC Jr, Lebailly F, Mantovani G, Mendonca LA, Garcia J, Liverneaux P. Telerobotic manipulation of the brachial plexus. J Reconstr Microsurg. 2012;287:491–4.
21. Miyamoto H, Leechavengvongs S, Atik T, Facca S, Liverneaux P. Nerve transfer to the deltoid muscle using the nerve to the long head of the triceps with the Da Vinci robot: six cases. J Reconstr Microsurg. 2014;306:375–80.
22. Facca S, Hendriks S, Mantovani G, Selber JC, Liverneaux P. Robot-assisted surgery of the shoulder girdle and brachial plexus. Semin Plast Surg. 2014;281:39–44.
23. Naito K, Facca S, Lequint T, Liverneaux PA. The Oberlin procedure for restoration of elbow flexion with the Da Vinci robot: four cases. Plast Reconstr Surg. 2012;1293:707–11.
24. Bruyere A, Hidalgo Diaz JJ, Vernet P, Salazar Botero S, Facca S, Liverneaux PA. Technical feasibility of robot-assisted minimally-invasive neurolysis of the lateral cutaneous nerve of thigh: about a case. Ann Chir Plast Esthet. 2016;616:872–6.
25. Guldmann R, Pourtales MC, Liverneaux P. Is it possible to use robots for carpal tunnel release? J Orthop Sci. 2010;153:430–3.

26. Tigan L, Miyamoto H, Hendriks S, Facca S, Liverneaux P. Interest of Telemicrosurgery in peripheral nerve tumors: about a series of seven cases. Chir Main. 2014;331:13–6.
27. Lequint T, Naito K, Chaigne D, Facca S, Liverneaux P. Mini-invasive robot-assisted surgery of the brachial plexus: a case of Intraneural Perineurioma. J Reconstr Microsurg. 2012;287:473–576.
28. Fleury M, Lepage D, Pluvy I, Pauchot J. Nerve transfer between the intercostal nerves and the motor component of the musculocutaneous nerve. Anatomical study of feasibility. Ann Chir Plast Esthet. 2017;62(3):255–60. https://doi.org/10.1016/j.anplas.2016.11.004. Epub 2016 Dec 29

Robotic Cleft Palate Surgery and Simulation

7

Dale J. Podolsky, David M. Fisher, Karen W. Wong Riff, Thomas Looi, James M. Drake, and Christopher R. Forrest

Abbreviations

DOF   Degrees-of-freedom
PSM   Patient side manipulator
RCM   Remote center of motion
TORS   Trans-oral robotic surgery

Introduction

Cleft lip and palate is one of the most common birth defects affecting approximately 1 in 700 births worldwide [1–3]. Cleft palate, where there is failure of fusion of the palatal shelves [1], requires surgical correction to ensure proper speech development, feeding, as well as minimization of social stigmatization. There are different techniques to repair a cleft palate, but they all share common principles: (1) closure of the oral side mucosa; (2) velar musculature re-approximation and reorientation; and (3) closure of the nasal side mucosa [4]. The procedure is typically performed around 1 year of age [4], before speech development begins.

D. J. Podolsky (✉) · D. M. Fisher · K. W. Wong Riff · T. Looi · J. M. Drake · C. R. Forrest
University of Toronto, The Hospital for Sick Children, Toronto, ON, Canada
e-mail: Dale.podolsky@mail.utoronto.ca; David.fisher@utoronto.ca;
Karenw.wong@sickkids.ca; Thomas.looi@sickkids.ca; James.drake@sickkids.ca;
Christopher.forrest@sickkids.ca

© Springer Nature Switzerland AG 2021
J. C. Selber (ed.), *Robotics in Plastic and Reconstructive Surgery*,
https://doi.org/10.1007/978-3-030-74244-7_7

The Challenges of Performing Cleft Palate Surgery

Cleft palate surgery requires operating within the small confines of the infant oral cavity using standard instruments with awkward orientations and trajectories while completing the required surgical steps. Visualization of the surgical field is suboptimal, and the tissues of the infant oral cavity are delicate, requiring precise dissections and tissue handling to ensure successful cleft palate closure [5]. In addition, adequate visualization of important anatomy during more radical dissections can be hindered [6, 7]. This is the primary reason that some surgeons use the operating microscope during cleft palate repair [8, 9]. This is compounded by evidence that surgeon experience [10, 11] and technique may impact patient outcomes. The procedure is also ergonomically challenging [12] requiring the surgeon to sustain awkward positions to access the palate. These features make cleft palate surgery technically demanding to perform as well as difficult to learn and teach.

The Potential Advantages of Using a Robot for Cleft Palate Repair

Robotic systems have been developed to overcome the limitations of performing surgery with standard and laparoscopic instruments. More dexterous and miniaturized instruments can perform surgery with less invasiveness and perform procedures that are not possible with existing instruments. Specifically, a surgical robot offers the advantage of improved visualization, access, precision, and ergonomics within confined difficult-to-access surgical workspaces [13, 14]. As a result of the unique procedural features of infant cleft palate repair previously described, cleft palate surgery is a suitable environment to take advantage of a surgical robot's enhanced capabilities.

Cleft Palate Simulator Test Bed

Surgical simulators can be virtual [15] or physical bench-top models [16]. Advantages of virtual models are the ability to provide scenario training [16] and the ease of obtaining objective performance metrics [15]. The advantage of physical simulators is the ability to simulate the constraints of a physical environment. Both virtual [17] and physical [18] simulators have been shown to translate into improved operating room performance. Several cleft palate simulators have previously been developed as both virtual and physical models [5, 19–22]. An appreciation of the confines of the infant oral cavity is critical to learn, and a physical cleft palate simulator provides an opportunity to perform a cleft palate repair using real surgical instruments.

A high-fidelity cleft palate simulator (Figs. 7.1, 7.2 and 7.3) has been developed and validated for the purpose of developing a robotic approach to infant cleft palate surgery [23] as well as for surgical training [24–26]. The cleft palate simulator allows performance of a complete end-to-end cleft palate repair procedure in a

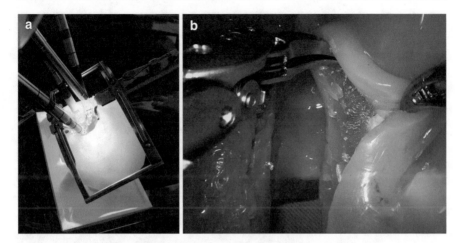

Fig. 7.1 (**a**) External view of the cleft palate simulator with three da Vinci robotic arms and an endoscope performing robotic cleft palate surgery. (**b**) Intra-oral view of a robotic approach to cleft palate repair using the cleft palate simulator during muscular dissection

Fig. 7.2 Intra-oral surgical view of the palate within the simulator after performance of a right lateral relaxing incision

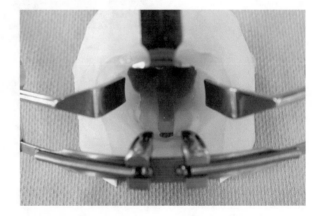

realistic physical environment. The simulator allows performance of the critical steps of cleft palate surgery (Table 7.1) using real surgical instruments while the user incises, dissects, handles, and sutures delicate synthetic tissue.

The cleft palate simulator has been evaluated as an effective and valuable training tool. Established techniques have been developed to evaluate surgical simulators. The traditional framework of face, construct, and content validity [27] is being replaced by the unitary framework proposed by Messick [28]. The central objective of this framework is to build sources of evidence supporting the simulator and its development process as being rigorous.

The simulator was developed using patient imaging, extensive computer modelling, three-dimensional printing as well as polymer and adhesive techniques to create a highly realistic simulated environment. Three expert cleft palate surgeons were

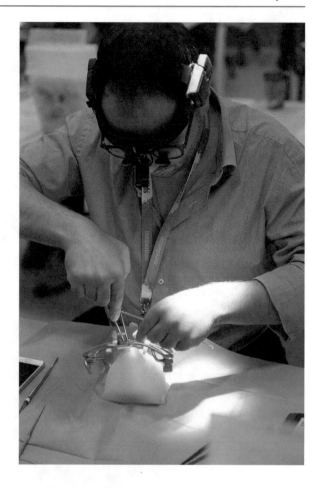

Table 7.1 Main steps of a cleft palate repair possible with the cleft palate simulator

1. Dingman insertion
2. Lateral relaxing incisions
3. Medial cleft margin incisions
4. Dissection of the oral mucosa from the hard palate
5. Dissection of the oral mucosa from the soft palate musculature
6. Release of the soft palate musculature from the posterior bony cleft margin
7. Dissection of the soft palate musculature from the nasal mucosa
8. Release of the nasal mucosa
9. Suturing the nasal mucosa together
10. Performing an intra-velar veloplasty
11. Suturing the oral mucosa together

involved in its design, and 26 experienced surgeons who performed a repair on the simulator found it to be realistic, anatomically accurate, and valuable as a training tool [24–26].

Use of the simulator has also been found to improve knowledge of cleft palate anatomy [24–26] and repair as well as improved procedural confidence [26]. An assessment of the learning curve using the simulator has been described using a newly developed and validated cleft palate specific objective assessment tool to assess technical performance. Repeated use of the simulator results in improved technical performance during simulated repair [24]. A hallmark of a valid simulator is the ability to stratify performance based on previous experience. A previous study found differences in performance among residents, fellows, and expert cleft surgeons using the simulator [24]. Electromagnetic sensors attached to trainees and cleft surgeon hands during simulated repair have demonstrated stratification of performance based on experience. In addition to its value as a training tool, its fidelity and accurate oral cavity dimensions make it a suitable environment to test robotic instruments.

Simulators as Test Beds for Developing Robotic Surgical Approaches

Infant robotic cleft palate surgery is currently at the experimental level. Given the implications to patient outcomes of technical error, it is helpful to investigate the feasibility of a robotic approach to cleft palate repair prior to testing on a real patient. This approach guides an understanding of design limitations for the development of more suitable systems without compromising patient safety. The utilization of surgical simulators for the development and testing of surgical instruments is an established method [29–31]. This approach provides a testing environment where the instruments can be pushed to their limits and where approaches can be more readily explored without compromising patient safety.

Trans-oral Robotic Surgery (TORS)

Trans-oral robotic surgery (TORS) using the da Vinci surgical system has become an established approach for adults, specifically for ablative procedures in head and neck surgery [32, 33]. Currently, the da Vinci remains the only FDA approved robot for performing TORS and can reduce morbidity for specific head and neck procedures compared to traditional approaches. However, the da Vinci surgical system was developed for multi-port procedures within large body cavities such as the abdomen and pelvis [34, 35]. The evolution of its use for trans-oral surgery was due to the lack of availability of more suitable systems for this specific application. Nonetheless, given the adoption of the da Vinci for TORS, investigating the feasibility of its use in the pediatric oral cavity is a suitable next step.

The da Vinci Surgical System

The da Vinci surgical system comprises a surgeon console (master) and patient side cart (slave) that contains four robotic arms (patient side manipulators (PSMs)), three of which couple to interchangeable EndoWrist instruments and the fourth to an endoscope (Figs. 7.4 and 7.5). The surgeon remotely controls the instruments and endoscope from the console. Each da Vinci arm has a remote center of motion (RCM) that is fixed in place (Figs. 7.4 and 7.5). This design feature was included to provide a fixed position along the instrument shaft where the instruments enter the body through a cavity wall (e.g., abdomen, pelvis, or thoraces), while the instruments are manipulated.

The typical setup during TORS comprises two instruments on either side of the endoscope triangulating through the oral aperture (Figs. 7.4 and 7.5). For TORS, there is a natural orifice through the mouth as opposed to a body cavity wall. Thus, the RCM is not necessary for TORS. As can be seen, the triangulation angles are acute, with the instruments and endoscope almost parallel to each other as they enter the oral cavity.

Perhaps the greatest technological achievement of the da Vinci is the design and function of the EndoWrist instruments (Figs. 7.5 and 7.6). The EndoWrist couples to the da Vinci arms (PSMs) and provides motion to miniaturized wrist mechanisms through steel cables. The wrist mechanism at the distal tip of the EndoWrist comprises multiple links that provides pitch, yaw, and grip motion. This allows for movement of a surgical instrument such as a scissors, grasper, or needle driver as well as a surgical blade, cautery, or dissector (instruments that do not require grip motion). Roll motion is provided at the proximal actuation mechanism adding to the

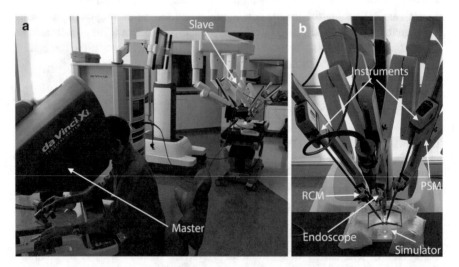

Fig. 7.4 da Vinci Xi setup for simulated infant cleft palate repair demonstrating (**a**) the master and slave setup and (**b**) two instrument arms on either side of the endoscope triangulating through the oral aperture

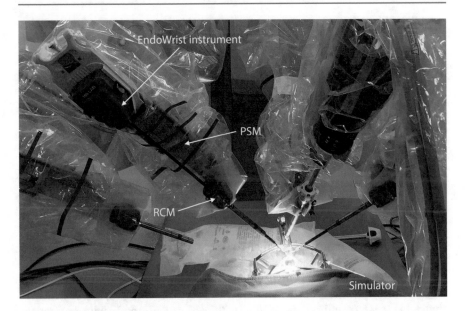

Fig. 7.5 da Vinci Si surgical system with EndoWrist instruments performing a simulated cleft palate repair using the cleft palate simulator

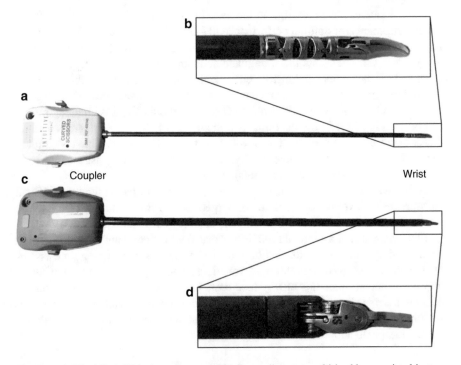

Fig. 7.6 da Vinci EndoWrist instruments. (**a, b**) 5 mm diameter multi-backbone wristed instruments. (**c, d**) 8 mm diameter pin-jointed wristed instrument

overall degrees-of-freedom of the system. The cable system allows miniaturization of the wrist mechanism by deporting the actuation system proximally at the level of the coupling mechanism (Fig. 7.6). In essence, a significant component of the mechanism complexity is proximal at the PSM where the EndoWrist couples to each PSM.

The Limitations of the da Vinci for TORS

The wrist mechanism provides three degrees-of-freedom (pitch, yaw, and grip) within a small workspace. This function allows articulation and performance of precise surgical maneuvers with more optimal instrument trajectories and angles within small body cavities. However, the instruments are large (5 mm and 8 mm diameter), and triangulating [36–39] a multi-port, multi-arm system through a single orifice results in frequent collisions between the arms and body as well as limitations in instrument excursion and manipulation [23, 36]. These limitations are present within the adult oral cavity workspace and are enhanced within the significantly smaller infant oral cavity. However, a small case series [40] and several case studies [41, 42] have utilized the da Vinci within the pediatric oral cavity. Limitations in the system and instrument design have prevented widespread use within the pediatric population [42].

Several studies have investigated the ideal orientation and positioning of the da Vinci instruments for optimal performance [37–39]. Sun and Yeung [38] performed an optimization method to determine recommended arm position and determined that (1) the instruments should triangulate at an angle of 45 to 90 degrees to each other and (2) the camera and instruments should form a triangle with the camera in the middle with a minimum distance of 5 cm from each other. These setup recommendations highlight why performing TORS with the da Vinci is challenging. As can be seen in Fig. 7.3, the instruments triangulate at less than 45 degrees and are closer than 5 cm to each other at the level of the trocar. This setup, which is required to visualize and access the palate is sub-optimal resulting in poor instrument excursion, manipulability, and frequent collisions.

A disadvantage of the da Vinci system is the absence of haptic feedback. Visual cues provide a level of feedback to the surgeon, but a true haptic system may be necessary to prevent excessive tissue forces that may cause injury.

Finally, the use of a surgical robot is associated with significant costs due to high capital and operating room expenditures as well as increased operating time associated with its use [43]. Adoption of robotic technology will hinge on whether improved patient outcomes may reduce costs enough to justify their use from an economic perspective. In addition, as more systems become available in the future with improved capability and efficiency, their use may become more palatable for more widespread adoption.

Robotic Cleft Palate Repair

Pre-clinical Studies

Two pre-clinical studies have investigated the feasibility of performing infant cleft palate surgery using the da Vinci surgical system [12, 23]. Khan et al. (2016) utilized a pediatric airway manikin to test the feasibility of performing cleft palate repair and pharyngoplasty using the da Vinci Si surgical system. They tested for optimal setup of the robot and found that the 0° endoscope was more suitable for cleft palate repair and that the 5 mm diameter instruments were optimal for the posterior pharyngeal wall [12]. Advantages of the robotic approach included improved maneuverability of the robotic system, as well as ergonomics for both the surgeon and the patient. Their conclusion was that da Vinci cleft palate repair and pharyngeal wall surgery are feasible.

Podolsky et al. (2017) tested the da Vinci Si with 5 mm instruments and the da Vinci Xi with 8 mm instruments for infant cleft palate repair [23] using the high-fidelity cleft palate simulator [24–26] previously described. In this study, a complete cleft palate repair from start to finish was performed using both systems and configurations comparing (1) robotic arm repositioning's required; (2) instrument-instrument collisions; (3) instrument-oral aperture collisions; (4) instrument excursion; (5) endoscope excursion; (6) ideal wrist orientation; and (7) visualization for each step of the repair. The da Vinci Xi with the larger 8 mm diameter instruments outperformed the da Vinci Si with 5 mm instruments. Use of the Xi resulted in no arm repositioning, fewer instrument collisions, greater instrument excursion, and more ideal wrist orientations during the procedure compared to the Si. Accessing the lateral extent of the hard and soft palate resulted in instrument-oral aperture collisions using the 5 mm diameter instruments.

These findings were attributed to the different EndoWrist design of the 5 and 8 mm instruments (Fig. 7.6). The 5 mm instruments have a multi-backbone snake arm mechanism that facilitates miniaturization at the expense of a longer mechanism length. The 8 mm instruments have a classical pin-jointed mechanism which requires more components, but has a shorter mechanism length. These design differences result in a greater clearance between the 8 mm instrument shafts with each other and oral aperture during surgical maneuvers compared to the 5 mm instruments and overall better performance.

However, for both systems, there were more limitations working within the posterior oral cavity (defined as surgical steps performed posterior to the level of the hard-soft palate junction). Advantages of the robotic approach included superior visualization, the ability to articulate the instrument wrist within the oral cavity, tremor reduction, ambidexterity, and ergonomics. These features provide the capability of more precise dissection and tissue manipulation. However, instrument-oral aperture collisions can be significant. Furthermore, the lack of haptic feedback provides no measure of preventing these collisions from potentially causing significant tissue injury. The conclusions from this study are that robotic surgery offers the potential to enhance precision and technique in cleft palate repair. However, the design of current systems need to be optimized for the specific and unique workspace requirements of the infant oral cavity.

Clinical Studies

The only clinical study that has been performed was by Nadjmi (2016) [40]. In this study, the da Vinci Si surgical system with 8 mm instruments was used to perform a component of the muscular dissection in 10 patients (mean age of 9.5 months) during cleft palate repair. The results were compared to 30 controls who had a traditional cleft palate repair. The robotic group had a longer procedure duration (122 vs. 87 minutes), but a shorter hospitalization (1 vs. 2.4 days). The author reported no complications. Advantages of the robot specifically discussed were superior ergonomics and visualization which facilitated careful identification and dissection of the palatal musculature. A disadvantage of the robotic approach was the absence of tactile feedback. Recommendations of smaller and more flexible instruments would enhance infant cleft palate repair.

Together, these studies demonstrate that a robotic approach to cleft palate repair provides specific advantages that may improve precision and technique that may ultimately lead to better patient outcomes. However, existing robotic systems require optimization and design modification to fully take advantage of the robot's unique capabilities.

Robotic Platforms and Instruments for Infant Cleft Palate Surgery

Overall System Architecture

The optimal system for trans-oral surgery has yet to be developed. As previously described, operating within the oral cavity requires all instruments and the endoscope to fit within a single orifice. Thus, a natural next question is whether a single-port system where the instruments and endoscope fit within one port may be more amenable for TORS or infant cleft palate surgery. Single-port systems can be classified as "X-type" or "Y-type" systems [44] and are shown for single orifice surgery in Fig. 7.7. The single-port systems have multiple instruments passing through a single port at a body cavity wall requiring only a single incision. For trans-oral procedures, the port is positioned within space (Fig. 7.7). X-type systems have multiple instruments crossing each other at the single-port level. Y-type systems have all instruments within a single shaft and have two configurations: undeployed where the instruments stay together and deployed where the instruments open up and spread apart.

Multi-port   **Single port**

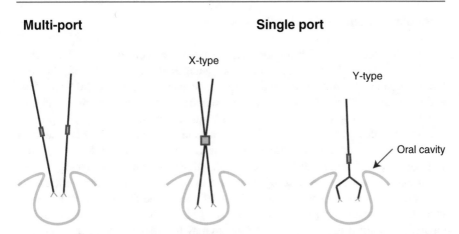

Fig. 7.7 Illustration of multi-port, X-type, and Y-type robotic single-port systems for TORS procedures. This figure was adapted from reference [44]

The clinically available single-port systems are the da Vinci Single-Site, which is an "X-type" single-port setup and the da Vinci SP, which is a "Y-type" system. The Single-Site system has been tested using the cleft palate simulator and was found to be incompatible with this particular workspace. Choi. et al. developed a similar system that employs an additional elbow joint intra-corporally that would likely improve instrument triangulation [45].

Several other Y-type surgical systems have been developed at the experimental level [46–50]. An interesting trans-oral specific system has been developed that is a permutation of the multi-backbone CardioARM. The mechanism comprises 50 cylindrical links that run in a follow-the-leader mechanism. Each link rotates ±10° from each other. The system has been tested in cadavers for laryngeal visualization and delivery of instruments and an endoscope [51].

The initial goal of single-port systems was to perform minimally invasive surgery through a single incision. However, for cleft palate surgery and TORS, there is direct access to the oral cavity. Thus, a single-port system may not be necessary and in some ways not advantageous, despite its perceived potential benefits. Single-port systems may impair manipulability within the oral cavity due to the large span of the instruments once they are deployed. The much anticipated da Vinci SP, which may appear to be a better option for trans-oral procedures, may in fact be more limited due to the position of its elbow joints.

The relative success of the previous feasibility testing for infant cleft palate repair using the da Vinci Si and Xi [12, 23, 40] may indicate that an optimization of the multi-port da Vinci type system may be more promising than the development or utilization of a Y-type system. The fundamental limiting factor for both the X-type and Y-type systems are the challenges of miniaturizing the instrument wrist while maintaining or enhancing the DOF required to perform complex surgical maneuvers.

Articulating Surgical Wrist Mechanisms

Articulation technology for robotic instruments varies considerably. Two review articles summarize the advantages and disadvantages of each type [52, 53]. Options include connecting rods, flexible structures, mechanical cables, fluidic actuators, and smart materials such as dielectrics and shape memory alloys. Fluidic actuators can be difficult to miniaturize. Dielectrics require very high voltages to provide necessary forces. Shape memory allows such as nickel titanium alloy are the most readily miniaturized, but are difficult to control. Mechanical cable designs can utilize continuum (5 mm EndoWrist) or pin-jointed (8 mm EndoWrist) configurations and are commonly used. As already described, the pin-jointed mechanisms are more difficult to miniaturize, but are more compact. Given the findings from Podolsky et al. [23] of better performance using the 8 mm instruments within the infant oral cavity, a miniaturized pin-jointed mechanism may be the most promising option.

Requirements for Infant Cleft Palate Surgery Robotic Instruments

Utilizing an understanding of cleft palate repair as well as available robotic systems and experimental designs, an optimal system design can be determined. The minimum number of DOFs to perform any general surgical step is seven (three position, three orientation, and one grip). Cleft palate surgery requires at least seven DOF given the unique shape and orientation of the palate. The instruments should be less than 5 mm in diameter and have a wrist with three DOF (pitch, yaw, and grip). The compactness of articulation should be minimized while providing maximum strength to perform surgical maneuvers. The system requires at least three robotic arms (ideally four) with two or three instrument arms and one endoscopic arm. More technical aspects of the design are that it minimizes internal friction to allow smaller cable calibers that aid in miniaturization. A summary of the design features can be seen in Table 7.2.

Many of the design requirements are met by the da Vinci surgical system. The missing component of the da Vinci is the existence of a more compact wrist mechanism that is less than or equal to 5 mm in diameter. Thus, development of a new wrist mechanism that couples to the da Vinci may be a suitable design enhancement that overcomes the current challenges of using the system for infant robotic cleft palate surgery.

New Instrument Design

A new wrist mechanism that has similar properties to the existing da Vinci 8 mm instruments was developed (Fig. 7.8) [54]. As previously described, the 8 mm instruments outperformed the 5 mm da Vinci instruments within the infant oral cavity due to its more compact articulation [23]. However, the trade-off is a more

Table 7.2 Design requirements for a cleft palate specific robotic system

System requirements
At least three robotic arms (ideally four)
One of the arms is an endoscopic camera for visualization
At least seven DOF
Wrist-specific requirements
Provides at least three DOF (pitch, yaw, and grip)
Diameter less than or equal to 5 mm
Compact articulation
Maximizes strength
Minimizes friction

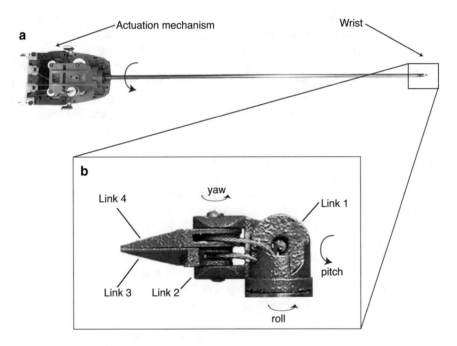

Fig. 7.8 (**a**) Newly developed wrist mechanism that has pitch, yaw, and grip motion (roll motion is controlled at the proximal actuation mechanism). (**b**) Link structure of the novel wrist mechanism and associated movements. This image was adapted from [54]

complex mechanism that is more difficult to miniaturize. The new wrist mechanism was 3D printed in stainless steel (Fig. 7.8). An EndoWrist was retrofitted with the new wrist mechanism that moves using steel cables that are driven at the actuation mechanism that couples to a PSM.

The new wrist design allows for further miniaturization at 5 mm diameter while maintaining the same DOF and reducing link lengths resulting in more compact articulation compared to the existing da Vinci 5 and 8 mm instruments. Specifically, the total length of the new wrist (from pitch to yaw axis) is 5 mm. The da Vinci 5 mm and 8 mm diameter designs are 9 mm and 16–19 mm in length. This results in greater clearance of the new instrument shaft from the oral aperture allowing for improved access to the palate and instrument excursion.

The new design incorporates cable guide channels (Link 1 in Fig. 7.8) eliminating the need for pulley's that add length and are difficult to miniaturize. However, the cable guide channels add friction to the system that increases cable tensions. Using an experimental setup, cable tensions increased from 0% to 37% when the wrist was pitched from neutral (0 degrees) to 90 degrees [54]. Maximum allowable cable tensions can be determined from the amount of tissue force encountered during cleft palate surgery. Preliminary investigation has determined that despite the increased friction due to the guide channels, the cable tensions are within the maximum tension thresholds for appropriately sized cables for this application. In addition, preliminary workspace analysis of this design demonstrates better fit within the infant oral cavity compared to the existing da Vinci instruments [54].

An additional challenge of this new wrist design is the changing cable circuit lengths as the wrist pitches. Novel articulation mechanisms are required to ensure constant cable tensions, and two proof-of-concept prototype systems have been developed that utilize either a spring or CAM mechanism [54]. The spring mechanism utilizes a spring to account for the changing circuit lengths. The challenge with this design is the inherent compliance of having a spring in series with the cables. The CAM mechanism (Fig. 7.8a) actuation mechanism) is more elegant and utilizes coupling between the wrist pitch and grippers to ensure cable circuit lengths are maintained during pitch motion. In essence, this new wrist design has reduced the complexity of the wrist mechanism at the expense of increased friction and increased complexity at the coupling actuation mechanism. The advantage of this trade-off is reduced size restrictions at the actuation mechanism facilitating miniaturization.

Further advancements in the novel wrist design described above have been developed [55]. Design modifications include an improved guide channel and CAM mechanism. Furthermore, the newer design modification was successfully prototyped, tested, characterized, and developed at 3 mm in diameter. This represents a significant evolution and breakthrough in pin-jointed wrist development.

Conclusions and Future Directions

Utilizing a surgical robot to perform cleft palate repair provides an opportunity to evolve the procedure to be more precise with the ultimate goal of improving patient outcomes. The da Vinci robot provides advantages such as improved visualization, access, precision, and ergonomics to a technically challenging procedure.

The cleft palate simulator provides a highly realistic platform to test existing and newly developed surgical instruments. As an approach to robotic cleft palate surgery evolves, the simulator will provide an opportunity to practice robotic cleft palate repair prior to operating on real patients. In addition to its use for testing instruments, the simulator provides a high-fidelity environment to practice traditional cleft palate repair techniques using standard instruments.

The pre-clinical [12, 23] and clinical [40] studies described using the da Vinci for infant cleft palate repair are promising. The pre-clinical studies provide the foundation for robotic system setup including optimal instrument positioning, orientations as well as the advantages and disadvantages of specific instruments for the infant oral cavity workspace. The only clinical study [40] available demonstrates that cleft palate surgery can be done safely in patients less than 1 year of age using the da Vinci. However, further developments are required to fully realize the robot's advantages. Existing instruments are large in size, and their design is sub-optimal for the infant oral cavity workspace.

Despite these limitations, the da Vinci platform architecture provides many of the requirements necessary for an infant cleft palate repair-specific system. A novel wristed instrument was designed and tested that couples to a da Vinci platform that features more compact articulation that is advantageous within the confines of the infant oral cavity.

The use of a surgical robot provides a platform for additional capabilities such as augmented reality [56]. Using high-resolution CT or MRI data, an overlay of critical structures such as blood vessels and nerves may be possible. Real-time perfusion scans that are currently available on the da Vinci [57] can be integrated to ensure that palatal flaps maintain their blood supply during more aggressive dissections.

As more surgical robotic systems are developed and evolved to smaller scales with more dexterity and capability, the equation of whether using a robot is advantageous swings in favor of its use. This equation will need to balance the robot's economic burden to the cost of complications that may require additional care and secondary surgery. Ultimately, the impact of using a robotic approach to cleft palate repair on patient outcomes will guide future use and widespread adoption among the global cleft care community.

Use of a robot in cleft palate surgery offers the opportunity to completely change how cleft palate repair is performed. The natural approach is to use the robot to emulate how the procedure is normally performed using standard instruments. However, a robotic approach should be developed from the ground up. For example, if instruments are developed with enough articulation capability at a small enough scale, it is within the realm of possibility that the nasal mucosa may be repaired from within the nose. This may offer a unique opportunity to more accurately and precisely repair the nasal mucosa. Similarly, there may be an advantage to repairing the velum and its musculature looking anteriorly from within the pharynx. This approach may provide a more accurate assessment of the muscular sling immediately after repair. Although these scenarios are hypothetical, their conception provides a framework for future research in this area that may fundamentally change the way cleft palate repair is performed.

References

1. Mossey PA, Little J, Munger RG, Dixon MJ, Shaw WC. Cleft lip and palate. Lancet. 2009;374(9703):1773–85.
2. Burg ML, Chai Y, Yao CA, Magee W, Figueiredo JC. Epidemiology, etiology, and treatment of isolated cleft palate. Front Physiol. 2016;6(67):1–16.
3. Woo AS. Evidence-based medicine: cleft palate. Plast Reconstr Surg. 2017;139(1):191e–203e.
4. Hopper RA, Tse R, Smartt J, Swanson J, Kinter S. Cleft palate repair and velopharyngeal dysfunction. Plast Reconstr Surg. 2014;133(6):852e–64e.
5. Vadodaria S, Watkin N, Thiessen F, Ponniah A. The first cleft palate simulator. Plast Reconstr Surg. 2007;120(1):259–61.
6. Sommerlad BC. A technique for cleft palate repair. Plastic Reconstr Surg. 2003;112(6):1542–8.
7. Cutting CB, Rosenbaum J, Rovati L. The technique of muscle repair in the cleft soft palate. Oper Tech Plast Reconstr Surg. 1995;2(4):215–22.
8. Sommerlad BC. Surgery of the cleft palate: repair using the operating microscope with radical muscle retropositioning–the GostA approach. B-ENT. 2006;2(Suppl 4):32–4.
9. Sommerlad BC. The use of the operating microscope for cleft palate repair and pharyngoplasty. Plast Reconstr Surg. 2003;112(6):1540–1.
10. Witt PD, Wahlen JC, Marsh JL, Grames LM, Pilgram TK. The effect of surgeon experience on velopharyngeal functional outcome following palatoplasty: is there a learning curve? Plast Reconstr Surg. 1998;102(5):1375–84.
11. Rintala AE, Haapanen ML. The correlation between training and skill of the surgeon and reoperation rate for persistent cleft palate speech. Br J Oral Maxillofac Surg. 1995;33:295–8.
12. Khan K, Dobbs T, Swan MC, Weinstein GS, Goodacre TE. Trans-oral robotic cleft surgery (TORCS) for palate and posterior pharyngeal wall reconstruction: a feasibility study. J Plast Reconstr Aesthet Surg. 2016;69(1):97–100.
13. Selber JC, Sarhane KA, Ibrahim AE, Holsinger FC. Transoral robotic reconstructive surgery. Semin Plast Surg. 2014;28(1):35–8.
14. Selber JC, Alrasheed T. Robotic microsurgical training and evaluation. Semin Plast Surg. 2014;28(1):5–10.
15. Willis RE, Gomez PP, Ivatury SJ, Mitra HS, Van Sickle KR. Virtual reality simulators: valuable surgical skills trainers or video games? J Surg Educ. 2014;71(3):426–33.
16. Kazan R, Cyr S, Hemmerling TM, Lin SJ, Gilardino MS. The evolution of surgical simulation: The current state and future avenues for plastic surgery education. Plast Reconstr Surg. 2017;139(2):533e–43e.
17. da Cruz JA, Dos Reis ST, Cunha Frati RM, Duarte RJ, Nguyen H, Srougi M, et al. Does warmup training in a virtual reality simulator improve surgical performance? A prospective randomized analysis. J Surg Educ. 2016;73(6):974–8.
18. Cosman P, Hemli JM, Ellis AM, Hugh TJ. Learning the surgical craft: a review of skills training options. ANZ J Surg. 2007;77(10):838–45.
19. Senturk S. The simplest cleft palate simulator. J Craniofac Surg. 2013;24(3):1056.
20. Nagy K, Mommaerts MY. Advanced s(t)imulator for cleft palate repair techniques. Cleft Palate Craniofac J. 2009;46(1):1–5.
21. Matthews MS. A teaching device for Furlow palatoplasty. Cleft Palate Craniofac J. 1999;36(1):64–6.
22. Devinck F, Riot S, Qassemyar A, Belkhou A, Wolber A, Martinot Duquennoy V, et al. Suture simulator - Cleft palate surgery. Ann Chir Plast Esthet. 2017;62(2):167–70.
23. Podolsky DJ, Fisher DM, Wong Riff KW, Looi T, Drake JM, Forrest CR. Infant robotic cleft palate surgery: a feasibility assessment using a realistic cleft palate simulator. Plast Reconstr Surg. 2017;139(2):455e–65e.
24. Podolsky DJ, Fisher DM, Wong Riff KW, Szasz P, Looi T, Drake JM, Forrest CR. Assessing technical performance and determining the learning curve in cleft palate surgery using a high fidelity cleft palate simulator. Plast Reconstr Surg. 2018;141(6):1485–500.

25. Podolsky DJ, Fisher DM, Wong KW, Looi T, Drake JM, Forrest CR. Evaluation and implementation of a high-fidelity cleft palate simulator. Plast Reconstr Surg. 2017;139(1):85e–96e.
26. Cheng H, Podolsky DP, Fisher DM, Wong Riff KW, Lorenz PH, Khosla RK, Drake JM, Forrest CR. Teaching palatoplasty using a high-fidelity cleft palate simulator. Plast Reconstr Surg. 2018;141(1):91e–8e.
27. Xiao D, Jakimowicz JJ, Albayrak A, Buzink SN, Botden SM, Goossens RH. Face, content, and construct validity of a novel portable ergonomic simulator for basic laparoscopic skills. J Surg Educ. 2014;71(1):65–72.
28. Ghaderi I, Manji F, Park YS, Juul D, Ott M, Harris I, et al. Technical skills assessment toolbox: a review using the unitary framework of validity. Ann Surg. 2015;261(2):251–62.
29. Arezzo A, Ulmer F, Weiss O, Schurr MO, Hamad M, Buess GF. Experimental trial on solo surgery for minimally invasive therapy: comparison of different systems in a phantom model. Surg Endosc. 2000;14(10):955–9.
30. Niccolini M, Castelli V, Diversi C, Kang B, Mussa F, Sinibaldi E. Development and preliminary assessment of a robotic platform for neuroendoscopy based on a lightweight robot. Int J Med Robot. 2016;12(1):4–17.
31. Strauss G, Koulechov K, Hofer M, Dittrich E, Grunert R, Moeckel H, et al. The navigation-controlled drill in temporal bone surgery: a feasibility study. Laryngoscope. 2007;117(3):434–41.
32. Ghezzi TL, Corleta OC. 30 years of robotic surgery. World J Surg. 2016;40(10):2550–7.
33. Selber JC. Transoral robotic reconstruction of oropharyngeal defects: a case series. Plast Reconstr Surg. 2010;126(6):1978–87.
34. Pugin F, Bucher P, Morel P. History of robotic surgery: from AESOP(R) and ZEUS(R) to da Vinci(R). J Visc Surg. 2011;148(5 Suppl):e3–8.
35. Hussain A, Malik A, Halim MU, Ali AM. The use of robotics in surgery: a review. Int J Clin Pract. 2014;68(11):1376–82.
36. Marcus HJ, Hughes-Hallett A, Cundy TP, Yang G, Darzi A, Nandi D. da Vinci robot-assisted keyhole neurosurgery: a cadaver study on feasibility and safety. Neurosurg Rev. 2015;38:367–71.
37. Li Z, Glozman D, Milutinovic D, Rosen J. Maximizing dexterous workspace and optimal port placement of a multi-arm surgical robot. IEEE International Conference on Robotics and Automation; 2011; Shanghai, China. p. 3394–9.
38. Sun LW, Yeung CK. Port placement and pose selection of the da Vinci surgical system for collision-free intervention based on performance optimization. Proceedings of the 2007 IEEE/RSJ International Conference on Intelligent Robots and Systems; 2007; San Diego, CA, USA. p. 1951–6.
39. Li G, Wu D, Ma R, Huang K, Du Z. Pose planning for robotically assisted minimally invasive surgery. 3rd International Conference on Biomedical Engineering and Informatics; 2010; Yantai, China. p. 1769–74.
40. Nadjmi N. Transoral robotic cleft palate surgery. Cleft Palate Craniofac J. 2016;53(3):326–31.
41. Carroll DJ, Byrd JK, Harris GF. The feasibility of pediatric TORS for lingual thyroglossal duct cyst. Int J Pediatr Otorhinolaryngol. 2016;88:109–12.
42. Wine TM, Duvvuri U, Maurer SH, Mehta DK. Pediatric transoral robotic surgery for oropharyngeal malignancy: a case report. Int J Pediatr Otorhinolaryngol. 2013;77(7):1222–6.
43. Mahida JB, Cooper JN, Herz D, Diefenbach KA, Deans KJ, Minneci PC, et al. Utilization and costs associated with robotic surgery in children. J Surg Res. 2015;199(1):169–76.
44. Cheon B, Gezgin E, Ji DK, Tomikawa M, Hashizume M, Kim HJ, et al. A single port laparoscopic surgery robot with high force transmission and a large workspace. Surg Endosc. 2014;28(9):2719–29.
45. Choi H, Kwak HS, Lim YA, Kim HJ. Surgical robot for single-incision laparoscopic surgery. IEEE Trans Biomed Eng. 2014;61(9):2458–66.
46. Xu K, Goldman RE, Ding J, Allen PK, Fowler DL, Simaan N. System design of an insertable robotic effector platform for single port access (SPA) surgery. IEEE/RSJ International Conference on Intelligent Robots and Systems; 2009; St. Louis, USA. p. 5546–52.

47. Lee H, Choi Y, Yi B. Stackable 4-BAR manipulator for single port access surgery. IEEE/ ASME Trans Mechatron. 2012;17(1):157–65.
48. Quaglia C, Petroni G, Niccolini M, Caccavaro S, Dario P, Menciassi A. Design of a compact robotic manipulator for single-port laparoscopy. ASME J Mech Des. 2014;136(10): 105001.
49. Piccigallo M, Scarfogliero U, Quaglia C, Petroni G, Valdastri P, Menciassi A, Dario P. Design of a novel bimanual robotic system for single-port laparoscopy. IEEE/ASME Trans Mechatron. 2010;15(6):871–8.
50. Abbott DJ, Becke C, Rothstein R, Peine W. Design of an Endoluminal NOTES Robotic System. IEEE/RSJ International Conference on Intelligent Robots and Systems; 2007; San Diego, CA, USA. p. 410–16.
51. Rivera-Serrano CM, Johnson P, Zubiate B, Kuenzler R, Choset H, Zenati M, et al. A transoral highly flexible robot: novel technology and application. Laryngoscope. 2012;122(5):1067–71.
52. Jelinek F, Arkenbout EA, Henselmans PW, Pessers R, Breedveld P. Classification of joints used in steerable instruments for minimally invasive surgery-a review of the state of the art. J Med Devices. 2015;9(1)
53. Catherine J, Christine RL, Micaelli A. Comparative review of endoscopic devices articulations technologies developed for minimally invasive medical procedures. Appl Bionics Biomech. 2011;8:151–71.
54. Podolsky DJ, Diller E, Fisher DM, Wong Riff KW, Looi T, Drake J, Forrest C. Utilization of cable guide channels for compact articulation within a dexterous three degrees-of-freedom surgical wrist design. J Med Devices. 2019;13(1)
55. Wu G, Podolsky D, Looi T, Kahrs L, Drake J, Forrest C. A 3 mm wristed instrument for the da Vinci robot: setup, characterization, and phantom tests for cleft palate repair. IEEE Trans Med Robot Bionics. 2020;2(2):130–9.
56. Pessaux P, Diana M, Soler L, Piardi T, Mutter D, Marescaux J. Towards cybernetic surgery: robotic and augmented reality-assisted liver segmentectomy. Langenbeck's Arch Surg. 2015;400(3):381–5.
57. Hellan M, Spinoglio G, Pigazzi A, Lagares-Garcia JA. The influence of fluorescence imaging on the location of bowel transection during robotic left-sided colorectal surgery. Surg Endosc. 2014;28(5):1695–702.

Robotic Microsurgery in Urology Private Practice: Advantages and Outcomes

8

Mohamed Etafy, Richard A. Mendelson, Ahmet Gudeloglu, and Sijo J. Parekattil

Introduction

Beginning with the first recorded use of a microscope during surgery in 1970, the performance of microsurgical procedures has become quite common in contemporary times. In fact, it is widely referred to as the "New Revolution" in surgical interventions [1]. In particular, the use of microsurgical techniques and tools in the performance of fertility treatment in males has become the standard. At present, the tools have evolved to the point of the DaVinci Robot – a robotic microsurgical treatment modality that makes use of multiple arms that are controlled by a robotic surgeon (Intuitive Surgical, Inc., Sunnyvale, CA). The current literature suggests that the use of robotic surgical modalities for fertility treatment in males is a safe and viable course of action [2].

The most recent DaVinci models incorporate a 3D view camera allowing for magnification of up to 15×. Three robotic arms are incorporated and are capable of an identical range of motion to a surgeon's hand. Wrist and finger dexterity allows for a range of motion up to 180° articulation and up to 540° of rotation. The surgeon is able to revolve the instruments and manipulate them more than an authentic human hand without the risk of human issues such as tremor, muscular exhaustion,

M. Etafy
Avant Concierge Urology & University of Central Florida, Winter Garden, FL, USA

Alazhar Faculty of Medicine, Asyut, Egypt

R. A. Mendelson
Keiser University Graduate School, Ft. Lauderdale, FL, USA

A. Gudeloglu
Hacettepe University, Ankara, Turkey

S. J. Parekattil (✉)
Avant Concierge Urology & University of Central Florida, Winter Garden, FL, USA
e-mail: metafy@miami.edu

© Springer Nature Switzerland AG 2021
J. C. Selber (ed.), *Robotics in Plastic and Reconstructive Surgery*,
https://doi.org/10.1007/978-3-030-74244-7_8

or cramping. This has allowed for the development of new techniques and enhanced surgical ability that is no longer bound by the limits of human anatomy. Additionally, issues that human beings experience such as tremors and the unscaled motion of human hands are mitigated through the use of ergonomic and comfortable interfaces between the surgeon and the DaVinci Robotic Microsurgical tool. It also reduces the need for a surgical assistant's presence in the room in order to serve as an additional arm or to make use of a third surgical tool such as an ultrasound probe or some other imaging instrument in order to provide additional information to the surgeon performing the operation [3].

Animal studies were conducted to examine the efficacy of the use of robotic-assisted laparoscopic procedures after the introduction of robotics in surgical procedures, and this was followed by human trials in order to ensure that surgeons planning to use assisted robotic microsurgery (ARM) techniques would be able to operate based on abundance of literature and research [4–6]. Contemporary times see surgical procedures and techniques continuing to evolve through ongoing research [7]. Specifically, the topics of male infertility and chronic testicular pain, as impacted by ARM techniques, are explored in this chapter through a meta-analytic review performed in accordance with the Cochrane Guidelines and Preferred Reporting Items for Systemic Reviews and Meta-Analyses (PRISMA). A literature search was performed in the MEDLINE, Pubmed, and Cochrane electronic databases for a period from the year 2000 to the present using a Boolean search for the terms male infertility, robot-assisted, and robotic. Literature selected for inclusion in the current meta-analytic review included retrospective as well as comparative analyses. In all, a total of 23 articles were included.

The boon of robotic-assisted microsurgical procedures from the surgeon's perspective is the fact that it has made many previously open or laparoscopic procedures easily performed from a minimally invasive surgical modality. This leads to decreased risk of infection, decreased recuperative time, and overall decreased risk with regard to the surgical process. As a result, men who would otherwise have refused treatment are more likely to elect to have procedures completed as opposed to leaving the root conditions such as infertility and hernia untreated.

Techniques to be discussed in this chapter include robotic-assisted microsurgical vasovasostomy (RMVV), or vasectomy reversal; robotic-assisted microsurgical varicocelectomy (RAVx); and robotic-assisted microsurgical testicular sperm extraction (micro-TESE).

Robotic Microsurgical Vasovasostomy (RMVV)

Chronic orchialgia after vasectomy, known as post-vasectomy pain syndrome, which is associated with fullness of the epididymis and pain with intercourse, can lead to a recommendation of vasectomy reversal for some patients [8, 9].

The use of RVMM for the reversal of previously performed vasectomy procedures is demonstrated to mitigate some of the potential "human error" from delicate procedures involving fertility. As demonstrated by Kuang, et al. [10], the use of a robotic microsurgical modality reduced tremor but was demonstrated to increase the frequency of issues such as broken sutures, bent needles, and loose stitches [10]. Also of note, there was not a significant difference in terms of decreased fatigue for surgeons, considered to be minimal for both the surgeons using RMVV and the more traditional microscope-assisted surgical procedure performed without robotic assistance. Both groups completed all procedures with fidelity and led to patency of the vas deferens suitable for male reproductive ability to be restored. Surgical times differed considerably, with the traditional microscope-assisted surgeons completing the procedure in a mean (M) of 38 minutes and the RMVV surgeons completing the procedure in a M of 84 minutes. While this difference in time is considerable, it is important to note that in cases in which tremor can adversely impact the outcome of the procedure, RMVV is recommended as it eliminates tremor as a factor. Also, as surgeons became more familiar with the RMVV modality, surgical time decreased without compromising the integrity of outcomes indicating that the surgeons experienced an ability to learn through experience; thus, improving operative time as well as expected outcomes of future patients [8].

As iatrogenic vasal obstruction is a potential adverse side effect of procedures such as inguinal hernia repair (range from 0.3% in adults to 0.8% in pediatric cases), the need to develop and use varied surgical techniques exists. The incidence of infertility after these repairs is believed to be a result of the inflammation and fibrosis that result from the surgical intervention itself. As the axiom goes, "inflammation causes pain." Although the likelihood of this is relatively small, it is important to know that the condition can be treated. Trost et al. [11] explain that the use of RMVV in cases of iatrogenic vasal obstruction leads to improved long-term prognoses for patients as a result of the robotic modality having greater ability to conduct surgical procedures in areas that are otherwise challenging to repair.

Gudeloglu et al. [12] have published outcomes for 180 vasectomy reversal procedures (106 RMVV, 74 RMVE) [8]. In their series, they reported a 97% and 55% success rates in RMVV and RMVE procedures, respectively. Median operative durations (skin to skin) were also reasonable with 120 minutes for RMVV and 150 minutes for RMVE. See Fig. 8.1.

Use of RMVV has improved the outcomes as noted by Fleming [2]. This may be partially attributed to the fact that the learning curve is shorter than traditional procedures and surgical modalities. In summary, robotic-assisted microsurgical vaso-vasostomy (RMVV) is demonstrated to be a viable surgical treatment modality to reverse vasectomy procedures in otherwise healthy males [11].

Robotic-Assisted Microsurgical Varicocelectomy (RAVx)

Lines of treatment for varicocele included robotic, laparoscopic, open surgical intervention, embolization of varicocele veins. Treatment of varicoceles linked with a treatment for pain in the groin/testicle area [13], but Tulloch [14] identified the link between presentation of varicocele and infertility treatment upon examination of 30 patients presenting with varicocele who also demonstrated compromised

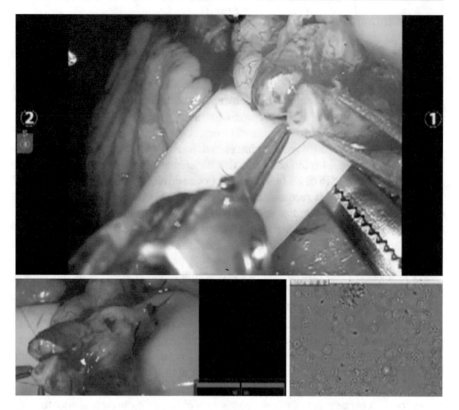

Fig. 8.1 Surgeon view on the surgeon console during robotic platform during robotic-assisted microsurgical vasovasostomy procedure

integrity of spermatozoa. According to Tulloch, these conditions presented in conjunction with a large percentage of patients demonstrating varicocele to some degree [14].

Varicocele correction is a staple in male fertility treatments, as varicoceles are credited as one of the most common causal factors in male infertility [15]. As such, there are a multitude of treatment options available in contemporary times including the open and laparoscopic varicocelectomy procedures. Research indicates that while the aforementioned options are feasible, microsurgical techniques yield more positive outcomes. As of the early 2010s, a major factor precluding robotic microsurgical intervention for varicocele treatment was cost; however, as robotic systems have become more widespread and the cost of such systems has decreased, robotic microsurgical treatment of varicoceles has become more commonplace, with the subinguinal microsurgical varicocelectomy becoming the standard treatment approach for varicocele [15].

The 1970s saw a zeitgeist in terms of the manner in which the world viewed microsurgery in a multitude of specializations. The first recorded instance of a microsurgical approach to varicocelectomy was not until 1985 when Marmar et al. [16] performed the first varicocelectomy using a surgical microscope and microsurgical tools. The outcomes of the microsurgical modality of treatment demonstrate improved semen parameters including concentration and motility [17]. In less than a decade, Marmar [18] had performed more than 600 of the microsurgical varicocelectomy procedures with a recurrence rate of less than 1% (0.82%). It was not until 2008 when Corcionne et al. performed the first robotic-assisted microsurgical varicocelectomy (RAVx) [19]. Barriers to widespread use of robot-assisted microsurgical varicocelectomy include the cost and availability of robotic microsurgical platforms. As stated earlier, with the passage of time, these issues have begun to correct themselves making RAVx more readily available to the masses.

Outcomes of the use of the RAVx procedure mirrored the outcomes of the microsurgical procedures, but costs were inherently lower, as use of the robot eliminated the need for a microsurgical assistant. Further, the data collected included outcomes from the very first performance of the involved surgeons using this procedure onward, which includes the learning curve. This means that as the surgeons become more comfortable and more fluid in terms of the RAVx skill set, outcomes are likely to eclipse those of the traditional microsurgical technique for varicocele correction [20]. See Fig. 8.2.

Our center reported the first use of a transscrotal approach for robotic microsurgical denervation of the spermatic cord and varicocelectomy. See Fig. 8.3. The outcomes appear promising. A better cosmetic result without groin pain might be a clinical benefit of this novel approach but further experience to fully evaluate its benefits and limitations is required. In 15 patients, 73% of the patients had a significant decrease in their pain within limited (median 3 months) follow-up time. Scrotal incisions healed with less scar than standard subinguinal incisions, and none of the patients reported numbness and pain in the incision site.

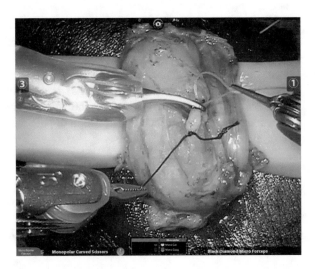

Fig. 8.2 Surgeon view on the surgeon console during robotic platform during robotic-assisted microsurgical varicocelectomy

Fig. 8.3 Transscrotal
varicocelectomy (Upper
image: transscrotal trocar
and robotic instrument
configuration, bottom
image: surgeon's view in
the surgeon console during
robotic-assisted
transscrotal
varicocelectomy)

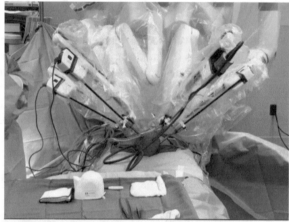

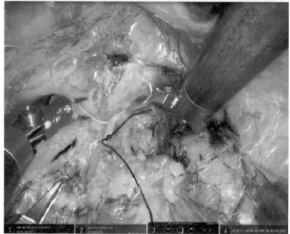

Microsurgical Denervation of Spermatic Cord

Chronic groin pain can be debilitating for patients. Microsurgical subinguinal denervation of the spermatic cord (MDSC) is a treatment option for this pain. Additionally, there are demonstrated psychological outcomes resultant from injury that can lead to castration such as perception of pain in that area [21].

Procedure

A robotic microsurgeon divides the structures that are known to house neural fibers without damaging arteries. These structures include the testicles, cremasteric muscle tissue, and deferential tissues. In an effort to reduce the occurrence of hydrocele,

Fig. 8.4 Surgeon view on the surgeon console during robotic platform during robotic-assisted microsurgical denervation of the spermatic cord

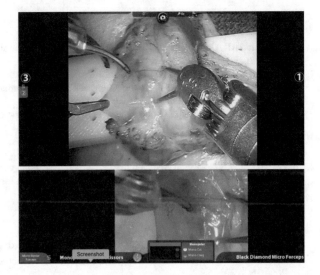

an effort is made to preserve lymphatic tissues. Further, the vas deferens is preserved in order to mitigate the manifestation of obstruction and fertility issues [9]. The justification for the use of this technique is that interruption of the neural pathway between the testicles/scrotal contents and the brain decreases afferent nerve tissue stimulation; thus, a decrease in reported pain issues is likely to occur. See Fig. 8.4.

In order to be considered a candidate for this procedure, a patient must have demonstrated positive outcomes to spermatic cord block. Work performed by Levine et al. demonstrated that a positive correlation exists between positive response to nerve block (>50% decrease in pain reduction) and permanent pain mitigation post MDSC [9]. Benson et al. demonstrated that men with a CO who demonstrate positive response to cord block demonstrate lasting and complete resolution of pain symptoms post MDSC [22].

Outcomes

Fifty patients evaluated by Marconi et al. demonstrated chronic scrotal pain. All of the 50 patients demonstrated positive outcomes when treated with a spermatic cord block while under local anesthesia. Pain was assessed using the Visual Analog Scale, or VAS. Six months post-operative date, 80% of patients reported complete mitigation of pain. An additional 12% reported persistent pain, and 8% reported no change in pain [23].

In our center, a retrospective review of 872 cases (772 patients) who underwent RMDSC evinced that over a median f/u of 24 months (1–70), 83% (718 cases) had a significant reduction in pain and 17% (142 cases) had no change in pain by subjective VAS scoring.

References

1. Lanfranco AR, Castellanos AE, Desai JP, Meyers WC. Robotic surgery: a current perspective. Ann Surg. 2004;239(1):14–21.
2. Fleming C. Robot-assisted vasovasostomy. Urol Clin North Am. 2004;31(4):769–72.
3. Parekattil SJ, Brahmbhatt JV. Robotic approaches for male infertility and chronic orchialgia microsurgery. Curr Opin Urol. 2011;21(6):493–9.
4. Parekattil SJ, Cohen MS. Robotic surgery in male infertility and chronic orchialgia. Curr Opin Urol. 2010;20(1):75–9.
5. Shu T, Taghechian S, Wang R. Initial experience with robot-assisted varicocelectomy. Asian J Androl. 2008;10(1):146–8.
6. De Naeyer G, Van Migem P, Schatteman P, Carpentier P, Fonteyne E, Mottrie A. Robotic assistance in urological microsurgery: initial report of a successful in-vivo robot-assisted vasovasostomy. J Robot Surg. 2007;1(2):161–2.
7. Parekattil SJ, Gudeloglu A. Robotic assisted andrological surgery. Asian J Androl. 2013;15(1):67–74.
8. Nangia AK, Myles JL, Thomas AJ. Vasectomy reversal for the post-vasectomy pain syndrome: a clinical and histological evaluation. J Urol. 2000;164(6):1939–42.
9. Adams CE, Wald M. Risks and complications of vasectomy. Urol Clin North Am. 2009;36(3):331–6.
10. Kuang W, Shin PR, Matin S, Thomas AJ Jr. Initial evaluation of robotic technology for microsurgical vasovasostomy. J Urol. 2004;171(1):300–3.
11. Trost L, Parekattil S, Wang J, Hellstrom WJ. Intracorporeal robot-assisted microsurgical vasovasostomy for the treatment of bilateral vasal obstruction occurring following bilateral inguinal hernia repairs with mesh placement. J Urol. 2014;191(4):1120–5.
12. Gudeloglu A, Brahmbhatt JV, Parekattil SJ. Robotic microsurgery in male infertility and urology-taking robotics to the next level. Transl Androl Urol. 2014;3(1):102–12.
13. Marmar JL. The evolution and refinements of varicocele surgery. Asian J Androl. 2016;18(2):171–8.
14. Tulloch WS. Varicocele in subfertility; results of treatment. Br Med J. 1955;2(4935):356–8.
15. Chan P. Management options of varicoceles. Indian J Urol. 2011;27(1):65–73.
16. Marmar JL, DeBenedictis TJ, Praiss D. The management of varicoceles by microdissection of the spermatic cord at the external inguinal ring. Fertil Steril. 1985;43(4):583–8.
17. Cho SY, Kim TB, Ku JH, Paick JS, Kim SW. Beneficial effects of microsurgical varicocelectomy on semen parameters in patients who underwent surgery for causes other than infertility. Urology. 2011;77(5):1107–10.
18. Marmar JL, Kim Y. Subinguinal microsurgical varicocelectomy: a technical critique and statistical analysis of semen and pregnancy data. J Urol. 1994;152(4):1127–32.
19. Corcione F, Esposito C, Cuccurullo D, Settembre A, Miranda N, Amato F, et al. Advantages and limits of robot-assisted laparoscopic surgery: preliminary experience. Surg Endosc. 2005;19(1):117–9.
20. Gudeloglu A, Brahmbhatt JV, Parekattil SJ. Robot-assisted microsurgery in male infertility and andrology. Urol Clin North Am. 2014;41(4):559–66.
21. Levine LA, Matkov TG, Lubenow TR. Microsurgical denervation of the spermatic cord: a surgical alternative in the treatment of chronic orchialgia. J Urol. 1996;155(3):1005–7.
22. Benson JS, Abern MR, Larsen S, Levine LA. Does a positive response to spermatic cord block predict response to microdenervation of the spermatic cord for chronic scrotal content pain? J Sex Med. 2013;10(3):876–82.
23. Marconi M, Palma C, Troncoso P, Dell Oro A, Diemer T, Weidner W. Microsurgical spermatic cord denervation as a treatment for chronic scrotal content pain: a multicenter open label trial. J Urol. 2015;194(5):1323–7.

Robotic Nipple-Sparing Mastectomy with Immediate Prosthetic Breast Reconstruction

9

Benjamin Sarfati and Samuel Struk

Introduction

Nipple-sparing mastectomy (NSM) is presently the reference technique in prophylactic surgery, and its indications in curative surgery are under evaluation. Nipple-sparing mastectomy is technically more complicated than skin-sparing mastectomy insofar as surgical exposure is more difficult. Choice of incision is consequently of paramount importance. Indeed, inadequate exposure can lead to incomplete excision [1]. Moreover, choice of incision is a key determinant of successful reconstruction. Any breast incision necessarily interrupts vascularization of the mastectomy skin flap and thereby increases the risk of skin necrosis and of nipple areolar complex (NAC) necrosis. This is particularly the case with hemi-periareolar incisions [1]. Difficulties in exposure are also liable to lead to prolonged use of retractors, thereby rendering more fragile the mastectomy skin flap and the risk of skin or NAC necrosis. And finally, some incisions are associated with deformation or secondary NAC dystopia; this is particularly the case with external radial [2] and hemi-periareolar [3] incisions.

Endoscopic nipple-sparing mastectomy has been developed [4–6] as a means of obviating these drawbacks. In clinical practice, however, due to technical constraints, this technique has never been adopted [4–7]. Indeed, the straight and inflexible surgical instruments used in are not suitable for use along the natural curves of the mammary gland.

Toesca et al. [8, 9] were the first authors to report on robotic nipple-sparing mastectomy (RNSM) with immediate prosthetic breast reconstruction. High-definition stereoscopic vision of the surgical site, motion scaling, and the improved dexterity provided by instruments with 7 degrees of freedom may overcome the difficulties

B. Sarfati · S. Struk (✉)
Institut Gustave Roussy, Villejuif, France
e-mail: benjamin.sarfati@gustaveroussy.fr

© Springer Nature Switzerland AG 2021

97

J. C. Selber (ed.), *Robotics in Plastic and Reconstructive Surgery*,
https://doi.org/10.1007/978-3-030-74244-7_9

encountered in endoscopy [9] and thereby enhance the oncological and aesthetic outcomes of NSM.

We have developed our own procedure of RNSM with immediate prosthetic breast reconstruction [10] which slightly differs from Toesca's. A prospective study has been conducted in Gustave Roussy to assess the feasibility, the safety, and the reproducibility of this procedure [11].

Advantages of Robotic Assistance in Nipple-Sparing Mastectomy

Nipple-sparing mastectomy is technically more demanding than skin-sparing mastectomy because surgical exposure is more difficult owing to the smallest incision. Difficulties in exposure are liable to lead to incomplete excision [1]. For instance, some authors have reported on the risk of incomplete excision associated with inframammary incisions [1]. Difficulties in exposure may also lead to prolonged used of retractors, which may damage the mastectomy skin flap and increases the risk of skin or NAC necrosis. Moreover, any breast incision necessarily interrupts vascularization of the mastectomy skin flap and thereby increases the risk of skin necrosis and of NAC necrosis. Finally, some incisions may affect notably the cosmetic outcome of the reconstruction. For example, the external radial and hemi-periareolar incisions are associated with deformation or secondary NAC dystopia [2, 3]. Choice of incision is consequently critical.

There are several advantages to performing a NSM under robotic assistance. First, robotic assistance ensures better exposure apt to facilitate oncological surgery as the gland is dissected under endoscopic vision. Second, a short incision located in the lateral thoracic region is used for this procedure. This incision is completely hidden by and under the patient's arm. More importantly, as there is no incision on the breast, surgical approach does not interrupt vascularization of the mastectomy skin flap. As a matter of fact, the risk of skin and NAC necrosis is reduced. Moreover, there is no risk of secondary NAC deformation of dystopia. And finally, as the scar is not under tension and located at some distance from the implant, the risks of scar disunion and implant exposure are also dramatically reduced.

Patient Selection

The intervention may be envisioned in all patients having an indication for NSM, with a cup smaller than or equal to C and presenting mild or moderate ptosis (stages I and II of the Regnault classification). In the event of big breasts or severe breast ptosis, robotic assistance will no longer be indicated, given the imperative need to decrease skin surface size (inverted T scar). On the other hand, a need to associate sentinel lymph node biopsy is not a contraindication insofar as it can be carried out by means of the same scar without robotic assistance.

Preoperative Drawings

The drawings are performed in standing position (Fig. 9.1). First, the footprint of the breast is marked. Then, the footprint of the bra is delineated. Finally, the incisions are drawn. A lateral-thoracic approach associates a high vertical scar of 3 to 4 cm, drawn from the superior border of the bra, with a low centimetric vertical scar, drawn 8 to 9 cm below the cephalad extremity of the previous incision. These incisions are located 6 to 7 cm posterior from the lateral-mammary fold. Rather than being left exposed in a visible area, the scars are thus hidden by and under the patient's arm. Mastectomy and reconstruction by prosthesis are performed using this approach. The higher scar enables the operator to introduce two trocars, to externalize the gland at the end of the intervention and, finally, to introduce the prosthesis allowing for immediate breast reconstruction. The lower scar is used to insert the third trocar and to externalize the drain at the end of the procedure.

Surgical Technique

Every procedure is performed with the da Vinci® Xi™ (Intuitive Surgical®, Sunnyvale, CA). The patient is placed in flat supine position with the robot at her head. The ipsilateral arm is first placed in 90° abduction on a surgical armrest for the non-robotic part of the procedure. Infiltration with a saline solution containing 1 mg/mL of adrenaline is used to reduce bleeding and to facilitate subcutaneous dissection of the gland. Subcutaneous dissection is then performed as far as possible with scissors (Fig. 9.2). Before inserting ports, one has to ensure that dissection is confluent between the two incisions in order to be able to insert the instruments under endoscopic vision. Then, the arm is placed above the head, with internal rotation and 90° abduction. This position reduces the conflicts between the arm of the patient and the robot. We have never experienced any brachial plexus injury with this position. The upper incision is closed and three 8-mm diameter ports are inserted. Robot docking is guided by the target sign, which has to be aligned both

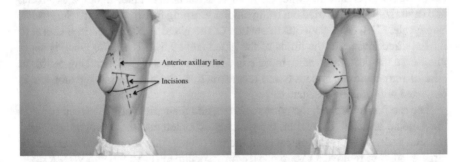

Fig. 9.1 Preoperative drawings. A lateral-thoracic approach associates a high vertical scar of 3 to 5 cm, located within the footprint of the bra, with a low centimetric vertical scar, located 8 to 9 cm below the previous incision. The scars are hidden by and under the patient's arm

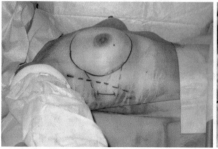
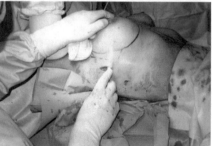

Fig. 9.2 Subcutaneous dissection of the gland is performed with scissors as far as possible in the crest of Duret plane

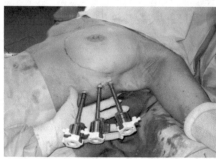
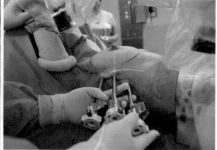

Fig. 9.3 Robot docking

with the skin incision and the nipple (Fig. 9.3). One port is connected to the gas insufflator to keep a constant pressure of 10 mmHg during the working process. Carbon dioxide insufflation creates an adequate working space for the robot (Fig. 9.4). The 30° camera (Intuitive Surgical®, Denzlingen, Germany) is introduced first in the middle port to allow non-traumatic insertion of the instruments under endoscopic vision. Dissection is performed with monopolar-curved scissors (Intuitive Surgical®, Sunnyvale, CA), whereas traction, counter-traction, exposure, and cauterization are carried out using bipolar grasping forceps (Intuitive Surgical®, Sunnyvale, CA). Subcutaneous dissection of the gland is completed in a lateral to medial direction, up to the limits of the gland (Fig. 9.5a). Then, the gland is separated from the pectoralis major muscle in a lateral to medial direction (Fig. 9.5b). In case of retropectoral implant-based reconstruction, the pectoralis major muscle is dissected with robotic assistance.

The robot is undocked, the ports removed, and the patient arm is placed back on the surgical armrest. Thereafter, the gland is extracted en bloc through the largest incision and sent for pathological examination (Fig. 9.6). A 4-cm incision is usually large enough to remove a C-cup mastectomy specimen (Figs. 9.6 and 9.7). A drain is placed through the inferior infracentimetric scar.

Fig. 9.4 Carbon dioxide insufflation. One port is connected to the gas insufflator to keep a constant pressure of 8 mmHg during the working process. Carbon dioxide insufflation creates an adequate working space for the robot

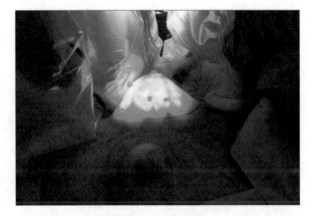

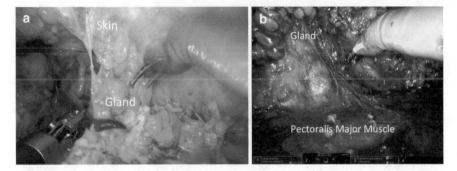

Fig. 9.5 Robotic dissection. Subcutaneous dissection (**a**) and prepectoral dissection (**b**) of the gland with the robot

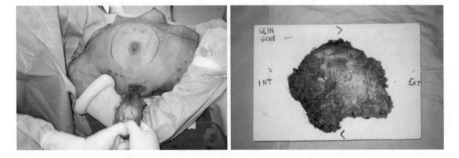

Fig. 9.6 Extraction of the gland. The gland is extracted en bloc through the largest incision. Example of a C-cup mastectomy specimen

Fig. 9.7 Final scar length
is less than 4 cm

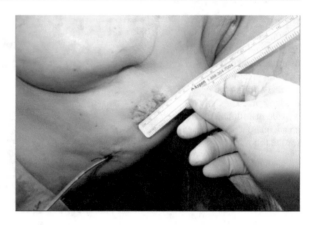

Breast reconstruction is usually performed with an implant in prepectoral position. Nevertheless, retropectoral reconstruction can be performed as well. The
implant pocket is closed laterally with two or three stitches between the skin and the
thoracic wall to avoid any secondary malposition of the prosthesis.

Results (Figs. 9.8, 9.9, 9.10, 9.11, 9.12, 9.13, 9.14, 9.15, 9.16, 9.17, 9.18, 9.19, 9.20, 9.21, and 9.22)

A prospective study has been conducted in our institution from November 2015
to July 2017 to assess the feasibility and safety of RNSM with immediate prosthetic
breast reconstruction. Sixty-three RNSM with immediate prosthetic breast reconstruction were performed in 33 patients (Fig. 9.7). There were no cases of mastectomy skin flap or NAC necrosis. We had to convert to an open technique in one case
(1.6%), which was the result of uncontrolled bleeding. Three infections occurred
(4.8%), one leading to implant loss (1.6%). No other major complications were
observed.

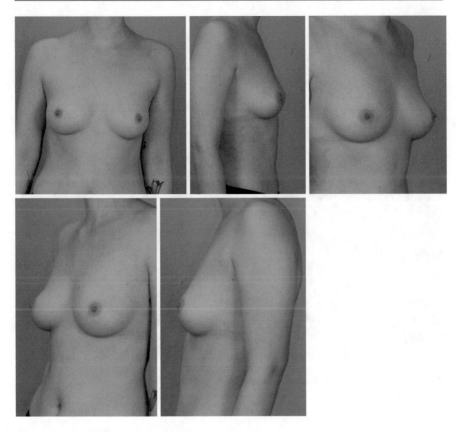

Figs. 9.8 and 9.9 Preoperative photos of patient A

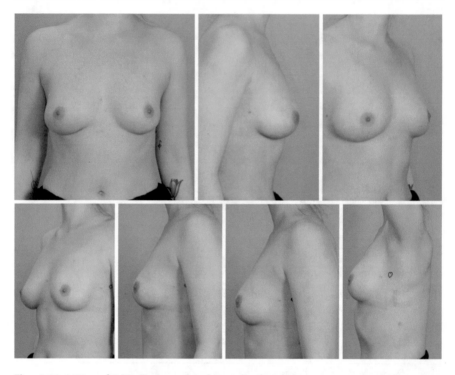

Figs. 9.10, 9.11, and 9.12 Postoperative photos of patient A

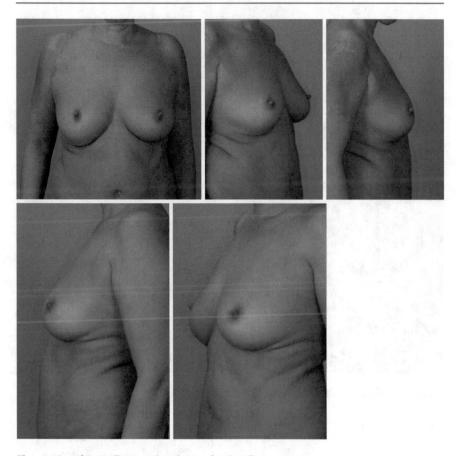

Figs. 9.13 and 9.14   Preoperative photos of patient B

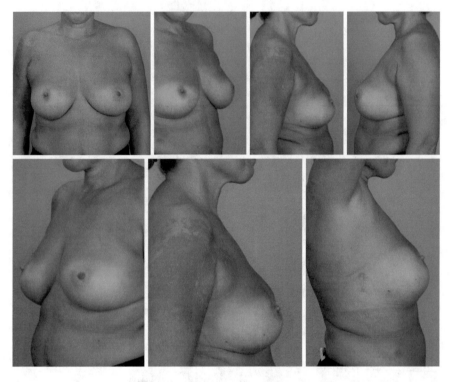

Figs. 9.15, 9.16, and 9.17 Postoperative photos of patient B

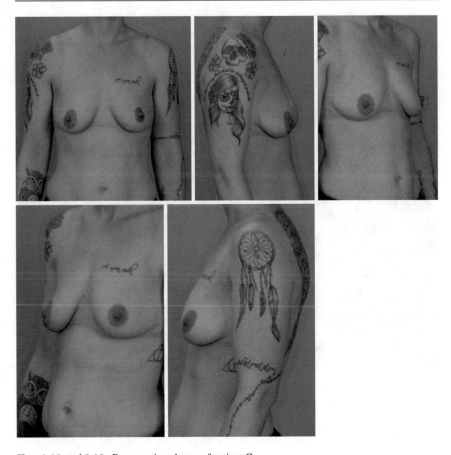

Figs. 9.18 and 9.19   Preoperative photos of patient C

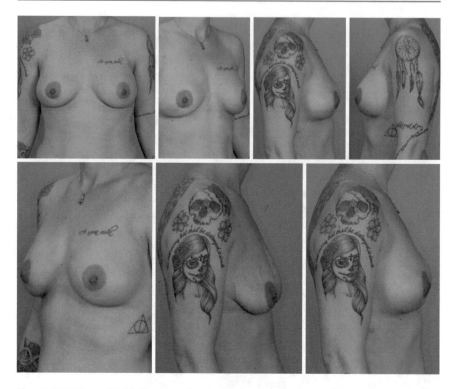

Figs. 9.20, 9.21, and 9.22   Postoperative photos of patient C

Conclusion

Advantages of this technique are a minimally invasive approach through a shorter and more acceptable scar and greater respect for the vascularization of the mastectomy skin flap. However, long-term data are needed to confirm the reduced rate of skin and NAC necrosis compared to the open technique, the oncological safety, and the aesthetic stability of the result.

References

1. Donovan CA, Harit AP, Chung A, Bao J, Giuliano AE, Amersi F. Oncological and surgical outcomes after nipple-sparing mastectomy: do incisions matter? Ann Surg Oncol. 2016;23(10):3226–31.
2. Wagner JL, Fearmonti R, Hunt KK, Hwang RF, Meric-Bernstam F, Kuerer HM, et al. Prospective evaluation of the nipple-areola complex sparing mastectomy for risk reduction and for early-stage breast cancer. Ann Surg Oncol. 2012;19(4):1137–44.
3. Choi M, Frey JD, Salibian AA, Karp NS. Nipple-areola complex malposition in nipple-sparing mastectomy: a review of risk factors and corrective techniques from greater than 1000 reconstructions. Plast Reconstr Surg. 2017;140(2):247e–57e.

4. Leff DR, Vashisht R, Yongue G, Keshtgar M, Yang G-Z, Darzi A. Endoscopic breast surgery: where are we now and what might the future hold for video-assisted breast surgery? Breast Cancer Res Treat. 2011;125(3):607–25.
5. Tukenmez M, Ozden BC, Agcaoglu O, Kecer M, Ozmen V, Muslumanoglu M, et al. Videoendoscopic single-port nipple-sparing mastectomy and immediate reconstruction. J Laparoendosc Adv Surg Tech A. 2014;24(2):77–82.
6. Lai H-W, Chen S-T, Chen D-R, Chen S-L, Chang T-W, Kuo S-J, et al. Current trends in and indications for endoscopy-assisted breast surgery for breast cancer: results from a six-year study conducted by the Taiwan Endoscopic Breast Surgery Cooperative Group. PLoS One. 2016;11(3):e0150310.
7. Ingram D. Is it time for breast cancer surgeons to embrace endoscopic-assisted mastectomy? ANZ J Surg. 2008;78(10):837–8.
8. Toesca A, Peradze N, Galimberti V, Manconi A, Intra M, Gentilini O, Sances D, Negri D, Veronesi G, Rietjens M, Zurrida S, Luini A, Veronesi U, Veronesi P. Robotic Nipple-sparing Mastectomy and Immediate Breast Reconstruction With Implant: First Report of Surgical Technique. Ann Surg. 2017;266(2):e28-e30. https://doi.org/10.1097/SLA.0000000000001397. PMID: 28692558.
9. Toesca A, Peradze N, Manconi A, et al. Robotic nipple-sparing mastectomy for the treatment of breast cancer: feasibility and safety study. Breast. 2017;31:51–6.
10. Sarfati B, Struk S, Leymarie N, Honart JF, Alkhashnam H, Kolb F, Rimareix F. Robotic nipple-sparing mastectomy with immediate prosthetic breast reconstructio n: surgical technique. Plast Reconstr Surg. 2018;142(3):624–7.
11. Sarfati B, Struk S, Leymarie N, Honart JF, Alkhashnam H, Tran de Fremicourt K, Conversano A, Rimareix F, Simon M, Michiels S, Kolb F. Robotic prophylactic nipple-sparing mastectomy with immediate prosthetic breast reconstruction: a prospective study. Ann Surg Oncol. 2018;25(9):2579–86.

Part III

Considerations for a Robotic Plastic Surgery Practice

Incorporating Robotics into a Plastic Surgery Practice

10

Alice S. Yao and Lars Johan M. Sandberg

Benefits of Robotic Plastic Surgery

Robotic-assisted surgery may still be fairly new to the field of plastic and reconstructive surgery, but some of its benefits may already be apparent to both new and established practices, including the improvement of patient outcomes, recruitment of new patients and referring physicians, attention of media or the parental institution, and broadening the surgeon's skills to prepare for the future.

It would certainly be enticing to any physician to have the opportunity to improve their patient outcomes. For example, robotic-assisted rectus abdominis harvest leads to decreased scar burden, pain, hospital stay, and return to work [1]. Not only could this benefit a physician's existing practice, but this prospect also means that a practice offering robotic surgery could increase its patient recruitment and new patient interest. Even if the interested patients turn out not to be candidates for the surgery, the availability of diverse procedures may make the physician's practice more desirable in a field of dense competition.

Similarly, the availability of technologically advanced procedures could be enticing to a new pool of referring physicians, particularly those who may be using robotic-assisted surgery in their own specialties. For example, if a colorectal surgeon is able to use robotic surgery to perform an abdominoperineal resection (APR) and therefore avoid a laparotomy scar, then it would be ideal if the reconstructive surgeon could also use a minimally invasive approach to perform reconstruction, for example, with a robotic-assisted pedicled rectus abdominis muscle flap. Even those

A. S. Yao (✉)
Division of Plastic and Reconstructive Surgery, Department of Surgery, Icahn School of Medicine at Mount Sinai, New York, NY, USA
e-mail: alice.yao@mountsinai.org

L. J. M. Sandberg
Oslo University Hospital, Rikshospitalet, Telemark Health Trust Skien, Norway,
Oslo, Norway

© Springer Nature Switzerland AG 2021   113
J. C. Selber (ed.), *Robotics in Plastic and Reconstructive Surgery*,
https://doi.org/10.1007/978-3-030-74244-7_10

referring physicians who do not perform robotic surgery may become more interested in a plastic practice that seems open to innovation and advanced procedures.

In addition to recruiting business from new patients and referring physicians, robotic surgery could bring attention to the plastic surgery practice in a broader sense. Media interest is often focused on innovation in medicine. Not only can surgeons attract outside interest to their own practice, but if they are affiliated with a hospital or academic center, then also to the parent institution. In those cases, there may be new opportunities for academic or financial promotion. If the hospital is supportive of innovation, then they may provide further support of the physician's technological pursuits in return, creating a synergistic and mutually beneficial relationship.

Finally, learning the robotic technique is an opportunity for any plastic surgeon to broaden his/her own perspective and learn new techniques. Plastic surgeons, in particular, should be malleable in an age of change and keep up with the demands of younger generations who may begin to seek their care. No practice should become stagnant, and new technology can push the surgeon to learn new skills and ways of thinking. Even if the robot is not practical for a particular surgeon's practice, understanding its indications is beneficial to any patient-physician discussion, and possibly even referral to another colleague if indicated. There is something honorable about offering the best care for a patient, even if it means losing a financial opportunity. Most importantly, learning new techniques and embracing technology mean that the plastic surgeon is more prepared for the ever-changing field of medicine. It may be possible to ignore these changes in the short term, but not in the long run as the surrounding world shifts its views.

Feasibility of a Robotic Practice (US Perspective)

Once a surgeon has decided that robotic surgery is an interest to pursue, it is important to consider whether it is practical to incorporate it into a plastic surgery practice. There are many factors to consider:

1. *Indication*

    Currently, the Da Vinci robot has seen applications to the field of plastic surgery through transoral head and neck surgery, muscle flap harvest (latissimus dorsi or rectus abdominis), and microsurgery/lymphatic surgery [2]. Emerging research includes robotic-assisted mastectomy and reconstruction [3, 4]. The future is limitless. However, prior to embarking on a commitment to such a large venture, the physician should have a clear idea of what kind of procedures will be in demand in the practice. This may be related to the surgeon's referral sources or patient population. For example, if one works with many otolaryngologists, then there may be a need for transoral robotic flap reconstruction. Alternatively, if the plastic surgeon has a large breast cancer population, then it may be useful to have the robotic-assisted latissimus dorsi flap as part of his repertoire.

Supermicrosurgery is one indication that may be an ideal concept for the robotic practice. The benefits are obvious with elimination of tremor and the motion scaling for operations on extremely small structures [5]. Lymphovenous anastomosis (LVA) is currently the most common supermicrosurgical procedure, and robotic LVA is in the process of making its way to the market (Fig. 10.1). However, the optics and instrumentation of the Da Vinci robot still require some development and optimization before it can be useful in a supermicrosurgical application. Other systems marketed overseas have expeditiously targeted this market with some success, but if the surgeon is planning on a US-based practice, then this would not be realistically accomplished at this time.

2. *Availability*

Depending on the location and type of hospital system in which the physician is working, access to a robot may be a limiting factor. The robot is of a price tag of $1–2 million US dollars [6], and therefore no physician newly entering the field would have the resources to acquire one individually. Therefore, most interested physicians would need to use one that is readily available in their hospital. While urban hospitals tend to have a higher quantity of these systems already in their institution, this does not necessarily mean that they are available for sharing. Large academic institutions have many urologists, gynecologists, and general surgeons fighting for time with the machines, and therefore may be restricted to a new physician requesting it. On the other hand, smaller community hospitals, if they happen to have a machine, may have one that is not fully utilized and may be happy to make better use of their investment with additional participants. This is highly variable at each institution and is up to the plastic surgeon to research the details. This can become even more complex if the new surgeon requires additional training prior to beginning practice, as he would then need to find a location where a robotic simulator is available.

Finally, it is not only the machine or equipment that is necessary, but also trained robotic operating room staff. Unless the hospital already has the staff readily available from their work with other departments (and are willing to share), the surgeon may need to train his own staff, or at the very least request

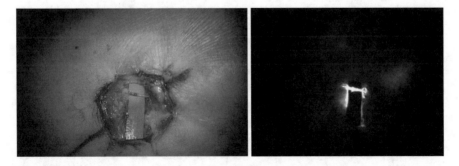

Fig. 10.1 A hand-sewn LVA of 0.7 mm with ICG passing through the anastomosis, a procedure suitable for future robotic microsurgery

representative support from the device company. It is important to note that often these companies will not offer support to non-FDA-approved procedures, even if the machine itself has been approved for use.

3. *Training*

Since robotic surgery is not an established sub-specialty within the field of plastic surgery, it is up to each individual surgeon to seek out training in this domain. This means that he would need to find an apprenticeship with one of the few established robotic plastic surgeons, or learn the technique on his own. This is much more difficult, as this would require not only access to a robotic simulator, but possibly also a robotic animal or cadaver lab in order to practice robotic skills prior to operating on live patients. Finally, it is important to keep in mind that no simulator can replace expert guidance, clinical experience, and feedback.

4. *Credentialing/hospital approval*

Similar to training, credentialing is quite tricky in this field due to the lack of established protocol. Factors to consider are both governmental regulations and institutional regulations. Smaller community hospitals may offer more flexibility in this case than larger academic centers, which have more regulations, administration, and red tape. In general, hospitals in the United States will require at the minimum: proof of machine proficiency (certificate offered by Intuitive Surgical), a case log of patients who have been operated on during training, and either fellowship certificate or other equivalent document from a proctor who can attest to the requesting physician's safety and efficacy using this technique. Alternatively, those physicians who are not able to learn through a mentor would need to apply for institutional review board (IRB) or investigative device exemption (IDE) approval in order to practice this technique on animals or cadavers prior to getting temporary privileges for patient interaction.

5. *Support*

Just because the hospital approves of the surgery, this does not mean that the system will support the physician's endeavors. Both administrators and other surgeons may see the robotic plastic surgeon as an inconvenience or even a threat to their current status quo. There is often pushback from other services utilizing robotic time, so the surgeon may need to search for other nearby facilities were the robotic time is not monopolized. Shockingly, one might even find resistance from his/her own plastics department, as older surgeons feel threatened by new technology and a competing practice that appears to be more advanced than theirs. Finally, the surgeon may even find negative feedback from their own institution despite bringing in positive publicity, due to pressure regarding utilization of equipment and financial resources.

6. *Financial*

The next most important question in feasibility is whether it is even *worth* it to add this endeavor to a plastic surgery practice. Note that in the United States, there is currently no robotic CPT code or modifier for plastic surgery cases, although this is likely on its way. The only option for additional reimbursement would be to use the code for "additional complexity" which is not always accepted by the insurance company. Therefore, there may be no additional financial compensation for performing this longer and more complex procedure on the professional fee side. If one is lucky enough to have a cash-only practice and willing patients, then this may be a worthwhile financial endeavor on a case-by-case basis. However, as mentioned above, the broadening of new prospects among patients, physicians, and institutions has an immeasurable price. On the technical fee side, ORs in which the robot is utilized are reimbursed at a higher rate than regular operating rooms. This means that the facility fees are higher in robotic surgery, translating into a higher hospital revenue. Depending on your hospital facility or system, this may make the contribution margin for a robotic procedure higher than a comparable open procedure.

7. *Time/perseverance*

   Since the robotic sub-specialty is still emerging within the field of plastic surgery, this endeavor is a massive undertaking. Interested parties will most likely encounter multiple obstacles on their way to learning the skill and achieving acceptance within their communities. Therefore, it would not be advisable for a clinician with limited time to dedicate to this. It would be best for those who are just starting their practices or who are willing to give up a portion of their established practice in order to cultivate the development of this fledging field.

Feasibility of a Robotic Practice (International Perspective)

The process of incorporating robotics into plastic surgery practice outside of the United States is in many ways similar to what is described above. Each country, culture, and system offers a unique set of practical and cultural challenges that should not be underestimated when deviating from old traditions and introducing new concepts. Some general aspects and perspectives on the challenges of building a robotic practice in a socialized system are as follows:

1. *Indication*

   In a socialized system, patient recruitment is different than in the United States. Referrals are based on diagnosis and hospital uptake area, and cannot be made to individual surgeons unless they are the only ones providing a specific treatment. Therefore, indication for whether to pursue robotics in plastic surgery is primarily up to the motivation of the plastic surgeon. Unlike patient recruitment, introducing a new procedure to the country in question does still take a significant amount of time and effort. One must prove the value of new techniques within the system. If the surgeon is exceptionally interested in starting a new technique such as robotic-assisted plastic surgery, he can start the approval process through research studies or efficacy/cost analysis (see section "Practical Approach to Starting the Robotic Practice" below).

2. *Availability*

   The acquisition of a robot can be a considerable expense. In certain settings, it may be easier to apply for research funds rather than ordinary healthcare funds to acquire a robot. If the surgeon is successful in motivating a consensus about the need for robotic-assisted plastic surgery, robot access is often provided by the hospital system. However, similar to the US situation, there is a competition between specialties in using the robot. Working together as part of another team and allowing more patients to benefit from minimally invasive surgery, such as is the case in robotic-assisted APRs, allow a fruitful cooperation rather than a competition.

Hospitals are in general required to keep their waiting lists for other "regular" procedures as short as possible or may otherwise be penalized. Operating room time is not as available in a socialized system. The number of hours is set and not very flexible. A longer waiting list or a longer procedure is thus not favorable for a socialized hospital. Therefore, when considering new technology, it is important to keep the procedure efficient.

In terms of equipment, there are many other machines available overseas than compared to the United States, where it is limited to a monopoly. At the University of Maastricht, the robotic LVA is currently being tested using the Microsure robot. Microsure (Holland) has developed a bolt-on system that utilizes optimal operating microscopes and allows the use of regular supermicrosurgical instruments. Medical Microinstruments (Italy) has developed a robotic system with specialized supermicrosurgical instruments. This system is also compatible with high-resolution microscopes and exoscopes. The commercialization of these systems will allow robotic LVA on a wide scale. These robots will likely not have many applications outside of plastic surgery, which decreases the competition for availability but requires the plastic surgeon or department to be financially responsible for the acquisition of these machines. Thankfully, the prices for these robots will likely be considerably less than for the Da Vinci system, favoring an expeditious commercialization process.

3. *Training*

Sound knowledge and experience is the foundation of any practice to provide safe and efficient surgery. As robotic plastic surgery is in its infancy, it is recommended to pursue a fellowship at a known robotic plastic surgery center or some other comprehensive training program to provide a solid foundation, regardless of whether practicing in the United States or overseas.

Robotic plastic surgery offers a mix of microscopic and laparoscopic surgery skills. Mastering these skills separately first is an advantage but not a necessity. In many countries, obtaining highly specialized training with the robot in other specialties than plastic surgery often requires joining a sub-specialty training program other than plastic surgery. This is not always easy to arrange for a plastic surgeon in training and may be considered a waste of time by program directors if the scholar is not intending to stay within the same subspecialty.

For many smaller and isolated countries, a lack of plastic robotic surgery centers means that training under a skilled plastic robotic surgeon as part of a microsurgical fellowship often is not possible without travelling abroad. An ECFMG certificate is required for a non-US resident to get a fellowship in the United States, and the preparations and efforts to obtain such a certificate are substantial and time consuming [7]. This certificate does not allow further practice in the United States beyond fellowship. A visa will also be needed as well as if planning a microsurgery fellowship match at a location that actually offers robotic plastic surgery [8].

4. *Credentialing/hospital approval*

When introducing an innovation such as robotic surgery in a socialized system, the focus is often on providing a consensus about the proof of overall benefit for the patient and comprehensively for the health system. The use of limited resources has to be justified. This is often done in a university setting, but it can also be done at a hospital with a strong academic and innovative background if the appropriate knowledge is present. In some countries, a formalized consequence analysis aiming for a 360-degree overview of the topic has to be performed and presented to the administration at the hospital in question. Efficacy of the method, cost, safety, ethical aspects, organizational consequences, training needs, staffing, evaluation of the current premises, current resources, need for investments, possible effects on other departments, patient logistics, number of patients who can benefit from the method, and new referrals from outside of the hospital's uptake region are all factors that are evaluated. A formal literature search has to be performed. The application goes through an independent peer review and also a review by an economic controller before a decision is made by the administration. This structured multistep evaluation process can be a valuable tool in that it offers a structured and clear path for the applicant. However, the process may be lengthy depending on the system. With fairly new methods that show promising results, but where the documentation is somewhat limited, it may be decided that an organized prospective research study may be called for.

The introduction of a new technique in a socialized system is not easy and requires a supportive and innovation-friendly environment. Willingness of the administration to make an investment in time and funds for the patients to reap the benefits of minimally invasive robotic surgery and robotic supermicrosurgery is crucial. The novel use of the robot must also not interfere with the hospital's compulsory activities. This may incur penalty fees for the hospital. A university hospital setting is often more favorable for innovation.

5. *Support*

A supportive environment on all levels is crucial. Having the support from a mentor to help start up a robotic program is an invaluable resource both for technical, cultural, and organizational issues. An external mentor, through his connections, may also facilitate the process of being welcomed in certain communities and cultures.

Another part of networking involves building the team that one will be working with in clinics and in the operating room. The dynamics of these relationships can be very different in different cultures. The experience of the authors is that involving the team in decisions and encouraging team input is always favorable and promotes the end goal. Nurses and operative technicians will have knowledge from procedures in different specialties that very likely can be applied to the plastic surgery procedure. Performing new surgeries that will revolutionize the field of plastic surgery often is associated with a steep learning curve, not only for the surgeon but also for his team. The operating time will initially be increased and at times "technological stand-still time" has to be expected. It is important to have the team onboard to prevent frustration at these times and to make the surgeries an exciting experience. This kind of "grass-root" support is important. Selber compares the team to a racing pit crew that can be a key part of the surgeon's success [2]. Work with a small team and choose dedicated staff if possible. Showing interest in the logistics of the procedure gives a greater understanding and also shows the team that the surgeon cares about all aspects of the procedure.

Finally, in modern socialized countries, patient-driven demands are generally handled by patient support groups; however, patient choice is more limited than in the United States. Patient support groups can be powerful allies in the process of introducing new techniques.

6. *Financial*

Socialized medicine also uses CPT codes to determine the allocation of funds to treatment and also to incentivize hospitals to provide efficient as well as high quality care. The individual surgeon, however, does not benefit from these codes. As an example, in Norway, the code ZXC 96 "Robot assisted procedures" is a modifier that increases the reimbursement by 29.3–58.6% for the procedure performed. This, of course, is a strong argument for management to support a robotic plastic surgery program.

In addition to the academic acclaim that comes from introducing a novel technique such as robotic-assisted surgery, the possibility of obtaining governmental or other research funds for the introduction of the technique also makes a good incentive for the management.

Practical Approach to Starting the Robotic Practice

Once the interested surgeon has committed to pursuing robotic-assisted plastic surgery, then he/she may consider the following steps:

1. *Learn the technique*

The easiest method is to find an apprenticeship through one of the few specialists in the world whose practice population matches up closest with the practice you are trying to build. Note that most plastic surgeons that participate in robotic-assisted surgery trend toward a narrow scope, such as either latissimus dorsi or rectus abdominis harvest. A secondary possibility is to find a robotic surgeon in a different field, such as urology or general surgery, as a mentor. While the procedures are not the same, a significant portion of the robotic technique is similar, including access and docking. If this were not feasible, then the surgeon would have to seek out a robotic simulator or laboratory. A robotic cadaver laboratory would be preferred, but these are also limited in location and may not be made available to "experimental" surgeons by the device company.

2. *Consider research*

Instigating a research project is a great way to introduce a new technique to a health care system. Developing new procedures may require that the initial efforts be evaluated in animal labs (with IACUC approval or similar) with a consequent progression to cadaver labs and later to full human operations. When looking for a place to practice robotic surgery, the presence of an animal lab with robotic competence and access to these resources represents a very valuable asset. As the research progresses to human trials, prospective randomized studies are preferable, but may be difficult to establish. In the early stages of a new treatment, simple observational studies are also of great importance and can lead the way for later prospective studies.

In addition to gathering data for the approval process, part of building an innovative practice is to document and share clinical results. A structured and well-thought-out plan from the start of a new practice will simplify later research efforts and improve their quality. Clinic and operative notes with a structured template can be beneficial for later retrospective studies. Keeping databases and registering data about patients comes with a great responsibility that should not be taken lightly, and often requires IRB approval. Internal audit is also of high importance in the beginning of the introduction of the new technique to provide the surgeon with feedback. Finally, peer reviews are not only of academic interest and self-improvement, but also of value for further building a practice. Today's patients are well oriented about the academic efforts of their surgeon.

If possible, one should strive toward getting grants from the state, universities, or other neutral funds, and not taking grants from the industry to avoid any conflicts of interest. However, when working with groundbreaking technology, any support and cooperation with a technology partner can certainly help to further the field. In these cases, all conflicts of interest should be clearly stated.

3. *Credential for patient care*

Once the technique is mastered and appropriate data presented, there are still restrictions to operating on live patients in most countries. If a mentor or fellowship is used, then the hospital usually requires an online certificate from Intuitive Surgical, a case log of patients, and a letter from the fellowship director/mentor validating the competence of the surgeon. If no mentor is involved, most institutions will require an experimental protocol to be approved prior to trying a new technique (see research section above). The surgeon would then be allowed to operate on a set number of patients and the results reviewed to assess for benefit versus harm. Once credentialing is obtained at one institution, particularly if a large and reputable one, then it may be used to support access at other surrounding hospitals as well.

4. *Network and build a team*

Assuming both the confidence and the credentials to practice are obtained, the next step would be to establish confidence in the community and the team. Surprisingly, newly invented procedures and recently minted surgeons are occasionally not welcomed with open arms in established communities. This may be due to more experienced surgeons not wanting competition, or due to support staff not wanting to learn new protocols. Nevertheless, it is the responsibility of the plastic surgeon to reach out to these colleagues and promote a positive relationship and hopefully circumvent any bitter sentiments. The first department to reach out to is the one that is currently using the robot the most in the hospital, as they will likely be territorial about their machine access. In most cases, this is urology. Others to consider are gynecology, general surgery, and otolaryngology. It may benefit the surgeon not only in the sense of getting approval for his endeavors, but also to cultivate a relationship for referrals. If colorectal surgery performs a robotic-assisted abdominoperineal resection, for example, then it would benefit the patient to also have a robotic-assisted perineal reconstruction.

Next, it is important to cultivate a relationship with the surgical support staff, that is, nurses and surgical technicians. They may need to be formally trained if not previously familiar with the process, or "borrowed" from another service that routinely performs robotic procedures. Either way, they would have to be notified of the necessary equipment and setup, which takes extra time for them to learn. It is crucial to go over this prior to actually performing the case for the first time. If the device representative is willing to participate (which may not be allowed for new procedures), then they are extremely helpful to the process, particularly for supplies, setup, and trouble-shooting.

5. *Advertise*

Once the plastic surgeon has a couple of successful cases under his belt, he may be interested in broadcasting the results to the local community. This could lead to benefits both in recruitment of new patients and referring physicians, and in proving to the hospital and community that this is a worthwhile investment. In a large institution, this is as easy as reaching out to the media department and asking for assistance. They can usually offer either a local institutional broadcast of print/electronic news, or utilize their connections with the outside media to promote a larger scope. If no organized media department exists, then the physician may need to personally call local radio or news stations to generate interest. Though this step is not crucial, it certainly is beneficial for the cultivation of a new technology.

6. *Balance finances*

Certainly, one would expect to operate at a financial loss for the first few cases due to longer times. However, this is not sustainable long term, so it is necessary to figure out the financial aspects of a robotic practice. In a hospital with a robot available for sharing, then the physician mostly has to worry about the robotic instruments, OR time, and staff. The robotic instruments are charged per-use, so it is advisable not to open or equip a certain instrument unless necessary to the case. However, it is also not advisable to use too few instruments if it causes inconvenience for the surgeon, because this would then increase operative time and therefore expense. This is where good planning comes in prior to surgery. The author usually prefers a grasper and a hot scissor to start a latissimus harvest, and a Maryland bipolar if needed for vessel ligation. Occasionally a surgical clip may be needed, but this could be done with a laparoscopic instrument instead of a robotic one. In general, the instrument count does not need to be excessive for most robotic-assisted plastic surgery procedures.

The next item to consider is the operative time. Robotic-assisted surgery has a sharp learning curve. The setup and docking time of the robot is often the largest obstacle. In breast reconstruction with latissimus dorsi, the muscle harvest time has been reported to average 1.5 hour with a range of 1–2.5 hours, as compared to an open technique of 1 hour [9]. The setup time does appear to decrease with experience. Again, preoperative planning and coordination with the team are crucial to a successful first few cases.

Unfortunately, at this time, there is no extra robotic code for the plastic surgeon. As mentioned above, in the United States one could try to use the −22 modifier for "extra complexity," which may or may not be accepted by the insurance company. Currently there is no immediate financial incentive to performing robotic-assisted reconstructions, unless the patients are willing to pay extra themselves. Many independent physicians, physician groups, or medical staff have built in agreements with the hospital that involve some type of revenue sharing. Given that technical charges are higher for the robotic cases, the well-organized and informed physician should be able to realize financial benefit from overall increased contribution margin of the case to the hospital.

Future Challenges

As if the challenge of training, credentialing, research, networking, and organizing finances were not enough, there are plenty of obstacles that may come up during the plastic surgeon's journey to achieve a robotic practice that have not been encountered as of yet. One could imagine litigation, equipment malfunction, competing technologies, and certainly others that we cannot even envision at this time. It is therefore important to maintain perseverance in all these circumstances, and keep in mind that those who do not embrace the future will fall behind!

References

1. Ibrahim AE, Sarhane KA, Pederson JC, Selber JC. Robotic harvest of the rectus abdominis muscle: principles and clinical applications. Semin Plas Surg. 2014;28:26–31.
2. Selber JC. Can I make robotic surgery make sense in my practice? Plast Reconstr Surg. 2017;139(3):781e–92e.
3. Toesca A, Peradze N, Galimberti V, Manconi A, Intra M, Gentilini O. Robotic nipple sparing mastectomy and immediate breast reconstruction with implant: first report of surgical technique. Ann Surg. 2017;266(2):e28–30.
4. Sarfati B, Honart JF, Leymarie N, Rimareiz F, Al Khashnam H, Kolb F. Robotic da Vinci Xi-assisted nipple sparing mastectomy: first clinical report. Breast J. 2017;24(3):373–6.
5. Hassanein AH, Mailey BA, Dobke MK. Robotic-assisted plastic surgery. Clin Plastic Surg. 2012;39:419–24.
6. Lee J. Surgical robot costs put small hospitals in a bind. Modern Healthcare. April 19, 2014. http://www.modernhealthcare.com/article/20140419/MAGAZINE/304199985.
7. Educational Commission for Foreign Medical Graduates. https://www.ecfmg.org.

8. American Society for Reconstructive Microsurgery. http://www.microsurg.org/fellowships/match.
9. Clemens MW, Kronowitz S, Selber JC. Robotic-assisted latissimus dorsi harvest in delayed-immediate breast reconstruction. Semin Plast Surg. 2014;28:20–5.

Part IV

New Microsurgical Robotic Platforms

Development of a New Robotic Platform for Microsurgery

11

Hannah Teichmann and Marco Innocenti

Robotic Systems for Microsurgery

While robotics has primarily penetrated laparoscopic surgery with the product offering of Intuitive Surgical Inc. and to a lesser extent orthopedic, spinal, and brain surgery with product offerings from Mako, Mazor, and Zimmer Biomet, plastic surgery has remained largely untouched by robotics to date, with the exception of a group of pioneering surgeons innovating surgery by attempting to reap the benefits of the da Vinci surgical robot outside of its indications for use [9]. In this section, we examine why existing robotic technologies do not fully cater to the needs of plastic surgeons, with a particular focus on reconstructive microsurgery, and how this technology gap has been attempted to be addressed by developing a robotic platform with wristed robotic microinstruments.

In the absence of a dedicated platform, the da Vinci Xi system has been used in open microsurgery procedures, including robot-assisted microvascular anastomosis [18]. The authors' suggestions for improvements to this system for microsurgical use mainly refer to the instrumentation, suggesting use of true microsurgical instruments, suitable for handling 9-0 or smaller sutures. In 2012, Maire et al. published the use of the da Vinci system for an exclusively robot-assisted toe-to-hand transfer [10]. An increase in operating time was explained by a lack of dedicated microsurgical instruments on the da Vinci system. The telemanipulator was reported to provide improved ergonomics and perceived higher precision through motion scaling. Nevertheless, the kinematics of the robot arms did not provide adequate precision, and the visualization system did not yield the same detail as a microscope [1]. Using

H. Teichmann (✉)
VP Clinical Development and Medical Affairs, MMI SpA, Pisa, Italy
e-mail: hannah.teichmann@mmimicro.com

M. Innocenti
Careggi University Hospital, Florence, Italy
e-mail: marco.innocenti@unifi.it

a da Vinci system to perform microsurgery requires modifying both workflow and OR setup. The potential of the use of robotics in microsurgery has hence been recognized by a number of surgeons and has driven the development of systems for this application as described below. Robotic tremor filtration, motion scaling, enhanced precision, and dexterity in tight spaces are some of the potential advantages to overcome manual limitations. There are ongoing and past academic research projects that have been launched to realize this potential. A number of prototypes have been developed for research purposes, with others having recently been brought to market by companies. A few examples and their design characteristics are described below.

Robotic assemblies for surgery or microsurgery comprising multi-joint robotic arms terminating with surgical instruments are known in the field. For instance, the surgical robot developed at the University of Calgary by Prof. Garnette Sutherland (document US-7155316-B2, known as NeuroArm) is a robotic assembly for performing MRI-guided brain microsurgery comprising an MRI-based image acquisition system and two multi-joint arms, each with three rotary joints with vertical axes to avoid direct gravity loads, each connected to its respective end-effector endowed with an internal degree of freedom (DoF) of motion for gripping [16].

The NeuroArm robot and many other solutions available in the state of the art, although offering partial advantages, require a motion strategy that simultaneously involves a plurality of independent movements even for small motions of the surgical instrument in the operating work-field, which results both in a difficult control of the kinematic accuracy and in a large encumbrance in the operating work-field, that in practice becomes inaccessible to the surgeon. The encumbrance of the surgical field and lack of dedicated instrumentation represent main technical limitations for robotic solutions for microsurgery. As a matter of fact, the application fields of the majority of robotic assemblies for surgery that are based on the teleoperation paradigm are dedicated to use in minimally invasive surgery (or MIS), such as laparoscopic or endoscopic surgery, as is the case for the da Vinci robot, where the dimensions of the anatomy provide more tolerance for large instrumentation and robotic arms. Currently, the da Vinci robot has approximately 5582 installed units and has performed around 1.2 million operations globally in 2019 (Intuitive company report 2019). In both endoscopic and laparascopic applications, the kinematics of the assembly is aimed to optimize the access of the surgical instruments to the operating field through the constraints of surgical ports or orifices, a feat that requires the coordination of a plurality of DoF of movement. In contrast, surgical, and microsurgical, applications in open surgery require an accurate kinematic control of direct translational movements, over a workspace limited by the field of view of the operating microscope.

The DoFs that are necessary for effective suturing must reflect the seven DoFs of the human wrist and grasping function, and have been validated by the wristed instrumentation of the da Vinci surgical system (EndoWrist). The execution of the principal surgical gestures, such as tissue tensioning and anastomotic suturing, requires the ability to orient the surgical instrument tip in a large spatial cone of directions and to rotate the instrument around its longitudinal axis (roll), for example to guide the needle through the tissue with the tip of the needle holder, in a similar manner as the human hand is jointed at the wrist and the elbow. Hence the seven DoFs can be described as three linear motions, roll, pitch, yaw and grasp.

Academically developed teleoperated robotic assemblies specifically for microsurgery have previously been described, such as the Robot-Assisted Micro-Surgery or RAMS developed at Caltech [5] and MUSA developed at the University of Eindhoven and subsequently by the spin-off Microsure [3]. These describe kinematic solutions for the movement of the surgical instrument tip that require coordination of a plurality of joints in a serial kinematic chain, which as a consequence visually encumber the operating field. The effect is increasingly pronounced as the joints articulating the tip of the instrument are further away from the tip itself. As a consequence, these microsurgical systems provide limited movement, and more specifically orientation, of the instrument tip when operating on a site within a limited cavity, such as 10 centimeters from the surface of the skin.

The RAMS system, pictured in Fig. 11.1, was created by NASA in collaboration with MicroDexterity Systems for microsurgical applications on the brain, eye, ear, and nose. It is a teleoperated system, where the two robotic arms are constituted by 6 DoFs that simulate the shoulder–elbow–wrist system with 3 axes of rotation. The master used by the surgeon is an exact replica of its kinematics. The RAMS platform was a very compact, versatile concept, which despite some potential benefits, was never commercialized, in part due to some fundamental limitations: the surgical tools are not miniaturized, and the instrumentation did not replicate the master movement with sufficient fidelity. The system has been tested in a preclinical setting, completing an end-to-end anastomosis on a rat carotid artery. The operating time was over twice the time required using a conventional approach [12, 15].

MUSA is a "Motion stabilizer" robot from the University of Eindhoven spinoff Microsure mentioned above, which uses manual microsurgical instruments mounted on robotic arms with six proximal DoFs, driven by master instruments mounted on the bedside. Similarly, the "Steady-hand" robot originally developed at Johns Hopkins University and currently under a license agreement between Galen Robotics and Johns Hopkins University uses mounted manual microsurgical

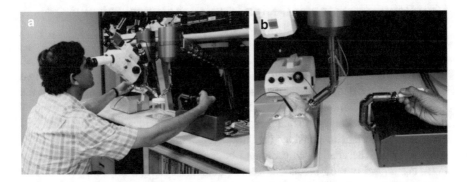

Fig. 11.1   RAMS Robot JPL. (Image Courtesy of NASA/JPL-Caltech)

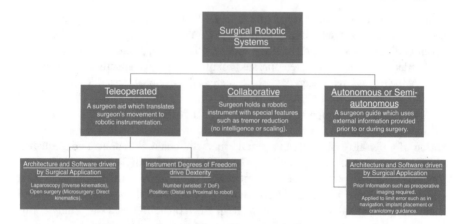

Fig. 11.2 Categories and characteristics of surgical robotic systems

instruments. The MUSA platform is a teleoperated platform in which the surgeon uses masters to drive the end-effector. The Galen robot uses a cooperative-control paradigm, and it is specifically designed to eliminate tremor by adding resistance to the surgeon's movement. The use of the Galen robot for anastomosis has been described in an ex vivo chicken thigh model [6]. While the use of the robot improved surgeon's tremor, it does not provide scaling of movement, which may be an important solution for increasing surgical precision through robotics in microsurgery.

The examples of innovations in surgical and microsurgical robotics named above allow us to categorize these devices as collaborative (e.g., Galen), semi-autonomous (e.g., Mako, Mazor), or teleoperated (e.g., da Vinci, MUSA). The latter may provide either distally wristed instrumentation (da Vinci) or non-wristed instrumentation (Musa). The type of robotic solution, architecture, instrumentation, and operating principle are driven by the clinical application with a value proposition toward error reduction, surgical access, tremor elimination, or precision. These categories are identified in Fig. 11.2.

User Requirements and Design Inputs for Microsurgical Robotic Systems

As the practice of microsurgery requires the use of either magnifying loupes, an optical or digital microscope, the practice demands a high level of dexterity and experience of the surgeon, who works at the limits of physiological tremor and the accuracy that human hand motions can reach at these dimensions. When considering opening the potential advantages of robotics to plastic surgery and microsurgery, it is important to consider that these procedures are performed in an open surgical field. The challenges presented here do not regard access to the surgical field, but regard motion precision, tremor, and scaling. With the exception of few innovative procedures that have harnessed the potential of laparoscopy to bring minimal invasiveness to plastic surgery, reconstructive procedures are open surgeries on an existing defect that are highly demanding from a manual standpoint in terms of precision required, but do not have the requirement of minimal invasiveness [7, 14]. These challenges of motion precision, tremor, and motion scaling define the user requirements and hence design solutions that an effective microsurgical robotic system shall provide to deliver increased precision. Increased precision is likely to require dedicated instrumentation as suggested by Willems [18].

The attempts at developing a dedicated robotic instrument for microsurgery described above address the main shift in concept of what robotic tools can offer to a surgeon. What a tool must offer depends upon the task at hand. The da Vinci system has offered access and dexterity to surgeons, and as a result, robotic surgery is frequently associated with improved access and the promise of increasingly less invasive interventions. The introduction of the distally articulated surgical instruments developed by Intuitive Surgical has manifested the advantage of having small movements at an instruments' tip for lending the surgeon precision in manipulating tissues and suturing without interfering with surrounding tissues, as occurs when the instrument's center of motion is more proximal to the robot.

In the case of microsurgery, the need is for dexterity and precision, potentially eliminating the effect of physiological tremor and easing the task. This requirement may be fulfilled by aggressive motion scaling and miniaturization of robotic instrumentation providing the appropriate DoF for surgical suturing. This type of solution could also find potential applications in transplant surgery, ophthalmological surgery, or in vascular surgery.

The primary roadblock to filling this technology gap is represented by the development of a miniaturized wristed robotic surgical instrument. Microsurgery requires high motion scaling for extremely small movements, with tremor reduction and instrumentation providing high precision and dexterity. This is ideally wristed instrumentation, which in the case of the small operative field, and the field of view under the microscope should not exceed the size of manual microinstruments or encumber the surgeon's view of the anatomy. The fundamental challenge of scaling wristed instruments to an appropriate size for microsurgery lies in the highly adverse scaling law that relates tip maximum force, tip stiffness, and precision with the instrument diameter.

It is clear that an engineering innovation is required to keep current instrument precision at an instrument OD of 2 or 3 mm, which is the instrument dimension deemed suitable for surgery under the microscope and required to match the dimension of current unwristed manual microsurgical instruments.

Medical instruments comprising a jointed device suitable for surgery are already on the market, primarily for the da Vinci platform. For example, the Intuitive Surgical EndoWrist is a robotic surgical instrument comprising a distally jointed device, capable of providing three degrees of freedom of motion, respectively, pitch, yaw, and grip, employing four actuation cables [2]. The cable-based technical solution for wristed surgical instruments limits the miniaturization of the robotic articulating device, as the pulleys do not lend themselves well to miniaturization and because friction created between parts limits the positioning precision achievable.

As the physical dimensions of an instrument are reduced, difficulties arise which are related to the increase of relevance of superficial forces, such as friction, that become dominant over volume forces. Such a phenomenon requires to resort to solutions that minimize friction forces, and at the same time reduce lost motion of mechanics to a minimum. The loss of positioning precision of an articulating device is a fundamental technological obstacle to further miniaturization of articulating. Moreover, the mechanical parts forming a surgical instrument wrist are very difficult to miniaturize below a 5 mm diameter using known fabrication methods, such as, injection molding and machining, and would be prone to have several locations of mechanical weakness. For this reason, current laparoscopic instruments have a shaft diameter or OD between 5 mm and 9 mm where only instruments with a 9 mm OD have a real gimbal wrist where the rotation is exercised around a single axis.

An attempt at miniaturization of the EndoWrist has been performed by Intuitive Surgical as described in US-2003-0036748-A1, which discloses a solution suitable for reducing the diameter of the surgical instrument to 5.1 mm [4]. This instrument foresees the use of a series of disks that function as vertebra, providing some flexibility; however, the bending of the instrument vertebrae cause an "elbowing" out of the wrist. Hence there is a trade-off between size and dexterity that has been made in previous attempts to miniaturize robotic instruments. The use of these two types of instruments in the plastic surgery scenario of pediatric cleft palate repair has underlined the trade-off described above and highlighted the need for a real miniaturized gimbal wrist for robotic plastic surgery [11]. In this study, a cleft palate simulator was used to compare the performance of the Si robot with 5 mm instruments to the Xi robot with 9 mm instruments. The performance was evaluated in terms of frequency of instrument-instrument collisions and instrument-anatomy collisions. The performance of the bona fide gimbal wrist of the Xi robot was superior to the "vertebrate" design of the Si 5 mm instruments, despite the larger diameter. However, the visual field is more encumbered in the case of the larger diameter instruments. The ideal solution would be one in which the instrument's radius of curvature is similar to its diameter, with a pivot-type joint, comprised of a pure axis of rotation.

These results highlight the importance of both dexterity and size of instruments for plastic surgery applications, which frequently represent constraints both due to the size and location of the anatomy. The surgeon may be presented with scenarios in which nerves or vessels are embedded in surrounding tissues, such as is the case in DIEP reconstructions either with axillary access to the thoracodorsal artery or intercostal access to the internal mammary artery. In this case, an articulation that is not at the instrument tip results in collisions with and potential trauma to surrounding tissue. Furthermore, an instrument with a 9 mm OD interferes with the visualization of the surrounding workspace the surgeon needs to take into account beyond point of contact of the instruments tips, given that the size of the typical working field of a surgical microscope can easily be around 10 mm in width or less when working at higher optical magnification that 15×.

A further obstacle to the miniaturization of jointed or articulated devices is the challenge of fabricating and assembling three-dimensional micromechanical parts with sufficient precision at a reasonable process cost. The need to develop relatively high forces at the tip in devices with a sub-millimeter size is very challenging even when dealing with suturing of "soft tissue" such as microarteries, veins, and nerves. In fact in order to grasp the needle firmly and drive the needle tip through the tissue, several hundred grams of force are required even when microsutures 9.0 or smaller are used.

Given the state of the art of surgical robotic interfaces and their end-effectors described above, there is hence a felt need for a surgical robotic assembly able to carry out precise motions and control a wristed medical instrument within a small surgical workspace using a simple driving method without compromising precision.

The criteria of tremor elimination and motion scaling, together with the experience of the benefits reaped from the EndoWrist's dexterity since the launch of Intuitive Surgical's product offering in 2000, have driven the development of a dedicated surgical robotic platform for microsurgery (Symani, MMI SpA). The requirements for such a product are high dexterity provided by a miniaturized wristed instrument, motion precision in the tens of micron range, tremor elimination, and extreme scaling appropriate for surgeons working at up to 40× visual magnification. Furthermore, surgeons must have the ability to switch between scaling factors based on the size of anatomy, magnification, and suture size and have a master design that allows for a rapid learning curve.

A small footprint in the operating room and sufficient mobility to allow movement between operating rooms are upsides as microsurgery is a technique shared by a number of surgical specialties, facilitating the logistics of sharing the technology between surgical units. End-user indications for a microsurgical robotic platform drove a surgeon-controlled, mobile platform with wristed robotic instruments suitable for microsurgery and the handling of sutures between 8-0 and 12-0 with appropriate tip force and grip force capabilities. Fulfilling these user requirements would redefine robotics beyond a tool enabling access and overcoming the cognitive hurdle represented by the inversion of movement around the fulcrum that a laparoscopic port represents, toward a tool-driving precision beyond manual capabilities. Current robots commercially available represent a technology gap in catering to microsurgeons both from a standpoint of the end-effector instrumentation and from a platform design standpoint.

The design and manufacturing of such surgical instruments and a robotic platform respecting these criteria have been innovated in a microsurgical robot which brings the instrument outer diameter down to 3 mm.

The wristed microinstruments are located at the tip of a 3 mm OD shaft, with closed jaws tip diameter of 0.3 mm, comparable with manual microinstruments. The kinematics of the instruments is based on the anatomy of the human hand and wrist, with 6 degrees of freedom for position and orientation, and 1 degree of freedom for grasping. Physiological tremor, known to be in the 100 μm range, is significantly reduced by scaling surgical movements by a factor of up to 20×, and by enabling positioning precision in the 10 μm range and motion steps of 1 degree [13]. The kit of microinstruments covers basic microsurgical instrumentation including dilator and needle holder and are suitable for handling 8-0 to 12-0 sutures (Fig. 11.3).

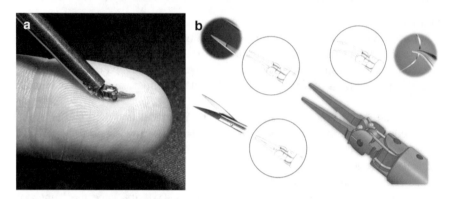

Fig. 11.3 MMI robotic instrument (**a**) and instrument kit design (**b**)

These instruments can be exchanged by a click-in system downstream of the sterile barrier. Furthermore, the microinstruments are mounted on shafts that are 12–15 cm in length, which should facilitate access in scenarios such as those described above (such as intraoral surgery, axillary, intercostal or other deep/far anastomoses).

These microsurgical instruments are mounted on a macropositioner arm that is passively placed over the operating field, under the operating optical or digital microscope (Fig. 11.4). Unlike laparoscopic robots that have multiple instruments that are placed independently, the instruments are hosted by a single arm and hence automatically placed in conjunction with each other, which relieves the operator of the burden of placing two separate robotic arms and instruments in such a way that they meet over the target anatomy. The robotic platform is independent of the vision system and can be combined with any magnification system that has a focal length of at least 25 cm, leaving space for the insertion of the macropositioner arm. The macropositioner arm itself is hosted by a cart, which can be brought to the bedside at the same time as the microscope, and allows easy movement within and between ORs (Fig. 11.4).

Using an optical operating microscope, the surgeon drives the robotic microinstruments by moving master instruments while looking through the eyepiece. In this scenario, the surgeon works within the sterile field, in an equivalent position and similar posture to traditional manual microsurgery. The switch between manual and robotic operating modes is immediate by manual removal of the macropositioner for safety or other reasons. Generally, even a specialized operator requires extended training to acquire mastery of the command devices adopted in known teleoperated systems. In fact, known master devices have a long learning curve, partially because they are mechanically anchored to motion recording stations, which necessarily limit the surgeons' movement in an unfamiliar way and often are of large dimensions. Hence, known master devices may be intrinsically unfit to replicate the function of traditional open surgery instruments and lack the ability to carry out a large spectrum of linear as well as angular movements in three-dimensional space, representing a limitation to the operator in learning the behavior of instruments in response to master input.

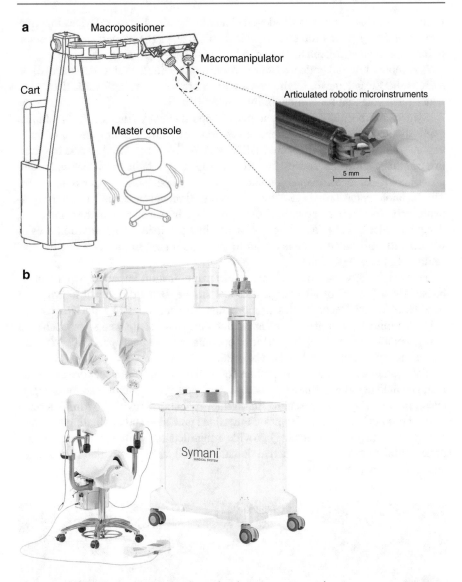

Fig. 11.4 MMI Microsurgical Robot Symani and components overview

Alternative approaches have been ideated to reduce such limitations. For example, a master control system developed by Intuitive Surgical (described in document US-8521331-B2, [8]) discloses a master worn by the surgeon as a glove on his or her fingers. A surgeon makes use of a display device integrated in the command device (console). This solution is partly advantageous, primarily from an ergonomic standpoint, but does not overcome the need for extended training before becoming proficient at handling the command devices instead of the familiar open surgery instruments. This has driven the development of handheld master devices that imitate manual surgical instruments in their shape, size, tactile properties, and method of handling by the surgeon as shown in Fig. 11.4.

A number of digital optical systems are currently being introduced to the market, such as the Zeiss Kinevo, Olympus Orbeye, Storz Vitom, and Novartis TruVision which have potential for compatibility with Symani.

Symani has been used both preclinically and clinically (Fig. 11.5). Preclinical application suggests safe and effective performance equivalent of superior of manual anastomosis (Marco Innocenti, BBM, and WSLS [19]). Clinical use has confirmed this, allowing successful free tissue transfer in post-traumatic and post-oncological reconstructions including the use of perforator-to-perforator flaps. This technology has proven effective in preclinical models and clinical use for lymphatic and vascular anastomosis, allowing for the adjustment to a dilating, pulsatile, dynamic structure (arterial anastomosis), and being able to cater to anastomoses of vessels with differing diameters or end-to-side suturing setups, maintaining the versatility of manual technique.

This technology for open surgery using magnification is part of what can be considered a "wave" of new surgical robots that are being developed to bring the benefits of robotic technologies to more surgical specialties beyond laparoscopy [17]. The miniaturization of mechanical and electronic components has enabled a new generation of lightweight platforms opening new surgical specialties to robotics and new procedures within these specialties.

The system described in this chapter fulfils the user requirements driven by the manual challenge represented by microsurgery, specifically, improved motion precision provided by motion scaling and tremor reduction provided by miniaturized wristed robotic instruments. By providing added precision and facilitating the practice of microsurgery, robotics may provide a significant contribution to overcoming undertreatment in the reconstructive domain as well as improve clinical outcomes and enable new procedures.

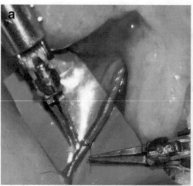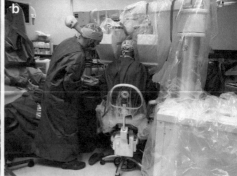

Fig. 11.5 Scenarios of preclinical (**a**) and clinical use (**b**) of Symani

References

1. Bouget D, Allan M, Stoyanov D, Jannin P. Vision-based and marker-less surgical tool detection and tracking: a review of the literature. Med Image Anal. 2017;35:633–54.
2. Burbank, WA. Four-cable wrist with solid surface cable channels. US 2010/0011901 A1. U.S. Patent and Trademark Office. 2010.
3. Cau R. Design and realization of a master-slave system for reconstructive microsurgery. Technische Universiteit Eindhoven. 2014. https://doi.org/10.6100/IR763107.
4. Cooper TG. Surgical tool having positively positionable tendon-actuated multi-disk wrist joint. PCT US2002/020884. World International Patent Office. 2002.
5. Das H. Tool actuation and force feedback on robot-assisted microsurgery system. US 6,233,504 B1. US Patent and Trademark Office. 2002.
6. Feng AL, Razavi CR, Lakshminarayanan P, Ashai Z, Olds K, Balicki M, Gooi Z, Day AT, Taylor RH, Richmon JD. The robotic ENT microsurgery system: a novel robotic platform for microvascular surgery. Laryngoscope. 2017;127:2495–500.
7. Ibrahim AE, Sarhane KA, Pederson JC, Selber JC. Robotic harvest of the rectus abdominis muscle: principles and clinical applications. Semin Plast Surg. 2014;28:26–31.
8. Itkowitz B. Patient-side surgeon interface for a minimally invasive, teleoperated surgical instrument. US20110118748A1. US Patent and Trademark Office. 2013.
9. Liverneaux PA, Berner S, Bednar M, Mantovani Ruggiero G, Selber JC. Telemicrosurgery. Springer Paris; 2012.
10. Maire N, Naito K, Lequint T, Facca S, Berner S, Liverneaux P. Robot-assisted free toe pulp transfer: feasibility study. J Reconstr Microsurg. 2012;28:481–4.
11. Podolsky DJ, Fisher DM, Wong Riff KWY, Looi T, Drake JM, Forrest CR. Infant robotic cleft palate surgery: a feasibility assessment using a realistic cleft palate simulator. Plast Reconstr Surg. 2017;139:455e–65e.
12. Saraf S. Robotic assisted microsurgery (RAMS): application in plastic surgery. In: Medical robotics. Rijeka: IntechOpen; 2008. p. 363–76.
13. Saxena A, Patel RV. An active handheld device for compensation of physiological tremor using an ionic polymer metallic composite actuator. In: In 2013 IEEE/RSJ international conference on intelligent robots and systems; 2013. p. 4275–80.
14. Selber JC, Baumann DP, Holsinger FC. Robotic latissimus dorsi muscle harvest: a case series. Plast Reconstr Surg. 2012;129:1305–12.
15. Siemionow M, Ozer K, Siemionow W, Lister G. Robotic assistance in microsurgery. J Reconstr Microsurg. 2000;16:643–9.
16. Sutherland GR (2006). Microsurgical robot system. US Patent 7,155,316. US Patent and Trademark Office.
17. Renaissance: a new generation of robots is about to enter the operating theatre. The Economist. 2017;425(9067):71–2.
18. Willems JIP, Shin AM, Shin DM, Bishop AT, Shin AY. A comparison of robotically assisted microsurgery versus manual microsurgery in challenging situations. Plast Reconstr Surg. 2016;137:1317–24.
19. Innocenti M, Menechini G, Malzone G. Robotics in super-microsurgery: making a more reliable and reproducible surgery. Barcelona: World Society of Lymphatic Surgery; 2020.

A Dedicated Robotic System for Open (Super-)Microsurgery

12

Ghufran Alshaikh, Rutger M. Schols, Joost A. G. N. Wolfs, Raimondo Cau, and Tom J. M. van Mulken

Introduction

Microsurgery is regarded as one of the most technically demanding surgical disciplines [1]. To perform microsurgical procedures, a significant level of experience is required, as well as the acquisition of great surgical skills. In microsurgery, accuracy is crucial for the quality and outcome of the procedure. This accuracy is limited by human capabilities, hence making this a prime area for the employment of robotics.

Robotic platforms offer potential advantages in the field of microsurgery. They are able to filter physiological tremor and allow for motion scaling (i.e., translation of large movements into sub-millimetric movements), thereby enhancing surgical precision. Robotic platforms offer better manipulation of instruments in smaller spaces that are difficult to be visualized due to challenging anatomy. Moreover, robotic assistance can reduce issues related to human fatigue by offering enhanced dexterity for its user, the surgeon [2, 3].

This chapter provides an overview of popular robotic platforms. Examples of robotic microsurgical applications in various surgical disciplines are elaborated. A new robotic platform that has been created especially for microsurgery at the authors' institution is presented (MUSA, Microsure B.V., The Netherlands). Current research on novel platforms for robotic microsurgery will be reported and future directions of robotic microsurgery are proposed.

G. Alshaikh
Maastricht University, Maastricht, The Netherlands

R. M. Schols · J. A. G. N. Wolfs · T. J. M. van Mulken (✉)
Maastricht University Hospital, Maastricht, The Netherlands
e-mail: tom.van.mulken@mumc.nl

R. Cau
Microsure, Eindhoven, The Netherlands

© Springer Nature Switzerland AG 2021
J. C. Selber (ed.), *Robotics in Plastic and Reconstructive Surgery*,
https://doi.org/10.1007/978-3-030-74244-7_12

Robotic Platforms

The Da Vinci system is currently the most commonly used Food and Drug Administration (FDA)-approved robotic surgical system (Intuitive Surgical Inc., U.S.A). Although initially designed for cardiac and laparoscopic applications, its potential advantages with regard to anatomical accessibility in microsurgery has been an area of interest. The system offers tremor filtration, scalable movements, 3-D visualization, and six-degrees of freedom. The use of novel adjunctive microsurgical tools has broadened the use of Da Vinci platform in the field of reconstructive microsurgery within several areas, such as plastic surgery, otology, neurosurgery, ophthalmology, and urology [4–7].

The Zeus system was also primarily designed for minimally invasive surgery. The system gained FDA approval but was later phased out from the market in favor of the Da Vinci platform. The Zeus system demonstrated to be able to perform microvascular anastomosis on rat femoral arteries. The end-to-end anastomosis were successfully performed and tremor minimization was noticeable by the surgeon [8].

These robotic platforms have been introduced into the medical field and provided new possibilities in a wide field of general surgical applications. However, none of these systems are especially designed to perform microsurgical procedures, and, therefore, they lack the requirements for real microsurgery. Currently, new robotic platforms are designed particularly for microsurgery.

In 2006, microsurgeons from the Maastricht University Medical Center (Maastricht, The Netherlands), performed a first robotic-assisted microvascular anastomosis in reconstructive microsurgery using the Da Vinci surgical system. This provided insight that robotic-assisted end-to-end microvascular anastomosis was feasible in the clinical setting and tremor minimization was noticeable [9]. Although the Da Vinci system offered great potential benefits in endoscopic procedures in many surgical specialties, the microsurgeons concluded that there were significant limitations of the system with respect to microsurgical procedures:

- The optics and magnification of the system were limited.
- The instruments of the device were large and powerful in relation to the delicate tissue and suture materials applied in microsurgery.
- The cost of disposables and relative complex operation setup was a drawback in clinical use.

On the other hand, the microsurgeons were convinced of the potential of robotic assistance in microsurgery, and this triggered these surgeons to search for a multidisciplinary collaboration for further development of robotic-assisted microsurgery.

A New Robotic Platform for Microsurgery

In 2007, a long-term collaboration was initiated between microsurgeons of the Maastricht University Medical Center and technical engineers of the Technical University of Eindhoven in the Netherlands with the main goal to overcome the limitations of existing robotic platforms by developing a novel robotic platform, especially for microsurgery.

The new concept involved a versatile solution compatible with current operating techniques, microscopes, and micro-instruments. The system is designed for high precision in open (super-)microsurgical procedures, and the design process was focused on the following: maximal surgical precision, safety, ease of use, cost efficiency, compatibility with existing microsurgical instruments and microscopes, and minimal changes in operation room setup and workflow.

In 2014, a first prototype of this new microsurgical robotic platform, so-called MSR Gen-1 (Microsure, The Netherlands) was created. The device assists microsurgeons by tremor filtration and motion scaling, thereby enhancing the precision of the surgeon and improving hand-eye coordination.

The system incorporates four main components:

A. Suspension ring
B. Master manipulators
C. Slave manipulators
D. Foot pedals

The surgeon controls forceps-like manipulators (master manipulators), which copy the surgeon's movement in real time to a micro-instrument held by the device (slave manipulators). The masters can be mounted to the operating table. The robotic slave arms are mounted to a suspension ring, which is placed between the operating field and the surgical microscope. This ring can be attached to the operating table. Up to four robotic arms can be used simultaneously and one or two operating surgeons can control them in a collaborative setup using the master manipulators. Figures 12.1 and 12.2 illustrate the different components and functions of the MSR.

Instrument accelerations and contact forces are deliberately minimized, and there is an ability to change motion-scaling settings in real-time using the foot

Fig. 12.1 Microsure's MUSA robot. Current generation of the first robotic platform for microsurgery

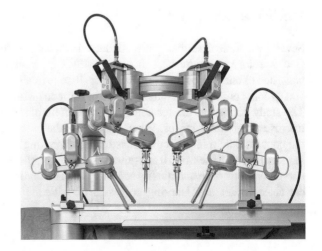

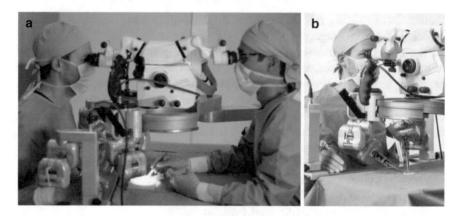

Fig. 12.2 (**a, b**) The operative setup of the Microsure microsurgical robot in a laboratory setting. (Re-printed with permission of the European Journal of Plastic Surgery, reference [11])

pedal. This provides the possibility of switching between very slow precise movements and quicker larger movements.

The size and weight of the system are small, enabling the surgeons and other staff to remain seated close to the patient and have direct view of the patient and the surgical site itself. The operation room setup can be maintained, saving costs and time. In case of device malfunction, the surgeon is able to promptly convert to manual continuation of the surgical procedure. The latter also makes hybrid operations an easy option: parts of the procedure can be performed manually while looking through the microscope, and when high precision is required, the robotic system can be incorporated. The system can be combined with any current or future camera system, making tele-surgery and incorporation of 3-D and virtual reality technology possible.

Preclinical Experience

Several preclinical studies were conducted to evaluate the performance of MSR Gen-1 prototype. Figure 12.3 shows the MSR Gen-1 setup in this study. One study consisted of anastomosing 2 mm diameter silicone tubes comparing robotic-assisted versus conventional micro-anastomoses of surgeons with variable level of expertise. The study confirmed the feasibility of the robotic platform to perform end-to-end microvascular anastomoses. When comparing the outcomes of robot-assisted with the conventional microvascular anastomoses, the time to perform these anastomoses was longer in the first 10 anastomoses. However, there was a very steep learning curve in robotic time and quality scoring [10]. The findings of adequate microsurgical anastomoses and learning curves in the silicone vessel studies were further

Fig. 12.3 Preclinical animal study using the first prototype of the Microsure microsurgical robot. (Re-printed with permission of the European Journal of Plastic Surgery, reference [11])

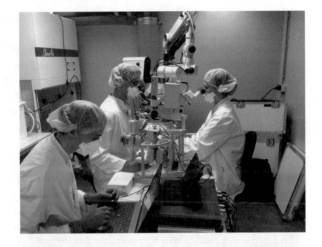

Fig. 12.4 Microsure MUSA robot holding genuine (super-) microsurgical instruments

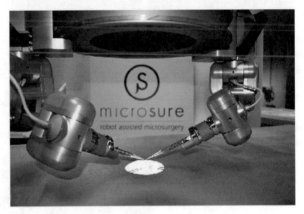

confirmed in an animal study in rats performing microsurgical end-to-end anastomoses of abdominal aorta and femoral arteries [11, 12].

First Commercially Available Robot for Microsurgery: MUSA

By encompassing the feedback of microsurgeons and taking lessons learned from the preclinical trials, a second-generation robotic platform, named MUSA, was created. The device was improved with solutions for sterilization, hardware maintenance, performance, and reliability. In addition, usability was improved regarding quick setup and removal of the system including an extended range of fine-tipped super-microsurgical instruments to be used in combination with the device as shown in Fig. 12.4. In 2019, CE-marking was achieved for the Microsure MUSA robot, making it the first commercially available robotic platform for microsurgery (Microsure B.V., The Netherlands).

First-in-Human Robot-Assisted Supermicrosurgery

A randomized controlled clinical pilot study, comparing robot-assisted lymphatico-venous (LVA) with manual LVA, was designed involving patients with early stage breast cancer-related lymphedema (BCRL). On September 01, 2017, microsurgeons at Maastricht University Medical Center performed the first clinical super-microsurgical intervention with the Microsure MUSA. Figure 12.5 shows the MUSA setup in the OR. The device was used to perform LVA on approximately 0.3 mm lymphatic vessels in the upper limb of patients suffering from BCRL. Evaluation at 3 months postoperative confirmed that it was feasible to complete super-microsurgical anastomoses in patients using the MUSA. Improvement in patient outcomes in terms of subjective complaints, quality of life, and arm volume were reported. The time to perform an anastomosis was longer in the robot-assisted LVA group; however, a steep decline in duration was seen during this trial [13]. Long-term results will be published after completion of this clinical trial.

Fig. 12.5 Robot-assisted lymphatico-venous anastomosis in a patient with breast cancer-related lymphedema using Microsure MUSA platform

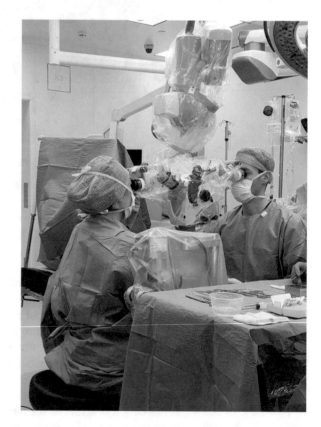

Other Novel Robotic Platforms

The use of robotic assistance in health care continues to grow as companies and health-care providers find innovative ways to use this technology to improve health care for patients. It is an active and growing research area, which is continuously overcoming critical challenges. Several other robotic platforms have been described for microsurgical applications. Chapter 11 also covers an example of a novel platform based on Da Vinci technology from our colleagues in the field.

Table 12.1 gives an overview of known robotic platforms with their currently explored surgical applications. Despite their acknowledged advantages, acceptance

Table 12.1 Overview of microsurgical robotic platforms currently under development

Platform (reference)	Institution	Explored microsurgical application(s)
Microsure MUSA[a] [14]	Microsure B.V. Eindhoven The Netherlands	Reconstructive microsurgery (e.g., lymphatico-venous anastomosis)
SPORT [15]	Titan Medical Inc., Toronto, Ontario, Canada	Not yet explored
RobOtol [16]		Otology (stapedotomy)
Eye Robot (version 2) [17]	Johns Hopkins University, USA	Ophthalmology (vitreoretinal surgery)
Preceyes[a] [18]	Preceyes B.V. Eindhoven, The Netherlands	Ophthalmology
Robotic retinal surgery [19]	University of Leuven, Belgium	Ophthalmology
Micron [20]	Carnegie Mellon University, Pittsburgh, USA	Ophthalmology: Membrane peeling (retinal surgery)
Smart surgical drill [21]	Brunel University, UK	Otology
Miniature Robot [22]	University of Bern, Switzerland	Otology
Bone attached robot [23]	Vanderbilt University, USA	Otology
µRALP [24]	Istituto Italiano di Tecnologia, Italy	Laryngology
REMS [25]	Galen Robotics, Inc., Sunnyvale, CA	Microlaryngeal phonosurgery
NeuroArm [26]	University of Calgary, Canada	Neurosurgery
MMI[a] [27]	MMI Srl (Pisa, Italy)	Reconstructive microsurgery
RVRMS [28]	Eye Hospital of Wenzhou Medical University	Ophthalmology
IRISS [29]	UCLA, Los Angeles, CA, USA	Ophthalmology
Da Vinci[a] [6, 7, 27, 30]	Intuitive Surgical (Sunnyvale, US)	Reconstructive microsurgery; vascular anastomosis;
Aesop [31]	Computer Motion Inc. of Santa Barbara, CA	Reconstructive microsurgery; Pedicle harvest
RAMS [32]	Jet Propulsion Laboratory (NASA, Pasadena, CA)	Reconstructive microsurgery; preclinical
EndoWrist [33]	Intuitive Surgical Inc.)	Urology

[a]CE approval

by the surgical community is one of the biggest challenges that these new platforms will face.

Robotic Microsurgical Applications

Modern microsurgery entails the use of high magnification, fine instrumentation, and microsurgical skills [34]. Currently, the Da Vinci system is the most widely used robot in the world. With its design for general endoscopic surgical procedures, the system poses limitations for microsurgical procedures. However, microsurgical applications using the Da Vinci system are increasingly being explored as described in Chaps. 1, 2, 3, 4, 5, 6, 7, 8, 9, and 10 of this book. The results of such efforts are not only contributing to establish clinical evidence of the benefits of robotics in microsurgery, yet increasing the interest of microsurgeons in robotic systems. This in turn generates positive feedback for the expansion of research into a wider range of microsurgical applications in other surgical fields. A general overview of robotic assistance is provided below.

Cardiac Surgery

Robotic-assisted microvascular surgery was first introduced in cardiac surgery in 1998 by Loulmet et al. after performing the first clinical computer-enhanced arrested heart coronary artery bypass using the Da Vinci system [35]. Few months later, Reichenspurner et al. repeated a similar procedure using the Zeus system (Computer Motion, Goleta, California, USA) [36]. In 1999, Boyd et al. performed endoscopic coronary anastomosis on porcine heart models using the Da Vinci system USA [37]. The same year this group also successfully performed a totally endoscopic beating heart bypass operation using the Zeus system [38].

Transoral Surgery and Otolaryngology

Transoral robotic surgery with the Da Vinci system has been performed in glottis microsurgery in a canine model [39]. The same system has been used in pharyngeal and micro-laryngeal dissections in cadaver models [40]. Transoral resection of the oropharynx in four patients with the Da Vinci robot was described by Ghanem et al. [4]. In otology, new robot-based microsurgical procedures were investigated to assist in performing middle ear microsurgery such as stapedotomy [41].

Ophthalmology

The utilization of robotic-assistance in ocular microsurgery has not progressed at the same pace as in other specialties. This is likely the result of the relatively large instruments of the Da Vinci system lacking the finesse and specific design for ocular microsurgery [42]. Nevertheless, robotic assistance has been demonstrated in vivo in amniotic membrane transplant and pterygium surgery [43]. In addition, robotic-assisted penetrating keratoplasty has also shown to be feasible using the new Xi Da Vinci system in experimental cases [42]. A novel robotic platform (Preceyes B.V., The Netherlands) is currently being evaluated in clinical setting for endoscopic intraocular surgery [44]. Compared with manual intraocular robotic surgery, the Preceyes robot showed fewer macular retinal hemorrhages and less intraocular instrument movement. Average time for the procedure was longer than the manual approach [18].

Neurosurgery

Robotic assistance has been reported in several neurosurgical procedures. Examples of clinical studies include brachial plexus repair and sympathetic chain repair to treat Horner's syndrome [2, 6, 45].

Urology

Robotic assistance has been widely used to tackle technically challenging urological procedures such as vasectomy reversal [46]. Additionally, these technologies are gradually becoming common place in male infertility procedures, e.g., vaso-vasostomy and vasoepidymostomy [33, 47]. Techniques and outcomes of other common andrological microsurgical procedures such as spermatic cord denervation and testicular sperm extraction have also been reported in the literature [48].

Plastic and Reconstructive Microsurgery

In 2005, the Da Vinci system was used to perform robotic-assisted microvascular anastomosis in a porcine free-flap mode [49]. One year later in 2006, Van der Hulst et al. successfully performed an arterial anastomosis for a muscle-sparing free TRAM-flap with the device [9]. In 2010, Selber reported the use of the Da Vinci system for reconstruction of oropharyngeal defects using a radial forearm, an anterolateral thigh flap and a facial artery myomucosal flap [50]. Maire et al. described a robot-assisted free hallux hemipulp transfer [7]. Furthermore, a conducted case-series detailing the use of robotic-assistance in latismus dorsi muscle harvest was published [51]. Progressively, demonstrations of rectus abdominis muscle and DIEP-flap harvest have been reported in literature [51–53], and is described in Chaps. 2, 4, and 5.

Super-Microsurgery

In 2010, the Society of Reconstructive Microsurgery defined the consensus on super-microsurgery: the technique of microneurovascular anastomosis for vessels of lumens less than 0.8 mm in diameter [54]. One of the main applications of super-microsurgery is in re-establishing lymph drainage via LVA for lymphedema treatment. The LVA procedure involves creating multiple bypasses between lymphatic vessels (0.3 to 0.5 mm in diameter) and subdermal venules (0.3 to 0.6 mm in diameter) [55].

At Maastricht University Medical Center, a first clinical trial was started to evaluate robotic-assisted LVA in patients with breast cancer-related lymphedema using the Microsure MUSA robotic platform [13]. Long-term results of this study will be published in the future.

Discussion – Future Directions

Future research should focus on further improvement of current robotic systems and novel robotic platforms for specific indications. Advances in software and mechatronics will allow surgeons to perform robotic-assisted microsurgical procedures with increasing precision and will also make new procedures possible. Multiple technical components will dictate the future of this revolution in (micro)surgery.

Lack of *haptic feedback* is often regarded as a disadvantage of robotic surgery. In microsurgery, visual cues can be used to mimic the perception of haptic feedback, even when true haptic feedback is absent. The lack of this feature in robotic-assisted microsurgery has been associated with micro-needle breaks, suture breaks during knot tying, and tissue laceration. The development and incorporation of haptic feedback in (super-)microsurgery would permit surgeons to feel extremely small forces that occur. This theoretical advancement will most likely improve surgical precision, tissue handling, and patient outcome as current manual super-microsurgery lacks haptic feedback.

Although robotic *tele-surgery* has already been proven feasible in general surgery in 2001 by operation Lindbergh, it is still not part of current hospital care. The likelihood for a surgeon to carry out microsurgery while located in a separate geographical location to that of the patient may become common practice in future microsurgery. A reliable connection without any lag is paramount to perform operations safely at a distance. Zhang et al. designed a robot for research and training in robot-assisted microsurgery with different interfaces for tele-surgery. A new hybrid tele-interface was introduced, in which position and velocity mapping are combined, thereby enhancing overall control efficiency [56].

Microsurgical instrumentation should be especially designed to meet the needs of the surgeons in terms of size and degree of articulation. Some microsurgical procedures demand specific micro-instrumentations to reach difficult anatomical regions, e.g., during reconstruction after resection of oropharyngeal tumors or during delicate ophthalmic procedures. The introduction of new instruments such as micro-doppler probes and hydrojet dissectors will further evolve and augment the surgeon's capabilities. Incorporation of biosensors on instruments could facilitate future guided super-microsurgery and early-stage intervention for malignancies at microscopic scales.

Optimal visualization of the surgical site is paramount during microsurgery. The development and incorporation of novel imaging modalities such as 3-D imaging, high-resolution stereotactic operation, spectral imaging, and real-time navigation systems are promising areas in the continued refinement of components of microsurgery. As technology continues to evolve, imaging tools are also likely to improve. Implementation of intraoperative visualization modalities such as Near-Infrared Fluorescence Imaging (NIRF) could facilitate real-time intraoperative anatomical navigation and contribute to critical decision-making [57].

Incorporation of *intraoperative image guidance* into the surgeon's console could also compensate for the lack of tactile feedback by providing additional visual cues that help improving the surgical efficacy. Perioperative use of ICG fluorescence is already considered to possess potential advantages for the assessment of anastomosis viability and monitoring of blood flow and tissue perfusion, thereby predicting the outcomes of reconstructive microsurgery [58].

The advantage of using a robotic device for microsurgical procedures is that any movement and force can be registered. This data can be used to enhance operative technique, provide microsurgical training, and standardize surgical outcomes. Assessment of microsurgical skills, which has traditionally been conducted by subjective observations of other trained surgeons, may eventually be replaced by objective assessment using standardized evaluation methods. Large data pools measuring parameters such as completion time, path length, depth perception, speed, smoothness, efficiency, bimanual dexterity, and forces measured can be applied to improve surgical performance in training and clinical care. These systems may provide effective and objective microsurgical training programs to produce microsurgical experts. *Cognitive surgical robots* are a new trend in the world of robotics that refer to intelligent robotic systems with cognitive skills and the ability of self-learning. Such systems are supported by surgical data science and are named as *big data analytics* which enables semi-automated surgery. The latter can help surgeons improve their operative procedures.

The interest in improving quality and efficiency in surgery extends beyond the operation table and translates to the pre- and postoperative experience: both for the patient and the surgical team. Online surgical data in combination with robot registration, calibration, and kinematic data will be a game changer in medicine. Extensive studies have suggested that collective surgical data from preoperative, intraoperative, and postoperative contexts provide accurate prediction of complications and could support surgical decision-making. This strategy is desired to reduce hospital costs associated with patients that have experienced complications.

Automation is also being considered as a potential tool for improved surgical workflow since the manual process can be time-consuming and does not provide direct feedback to surgeons for effective learning and enhancement of techniques. The authors expect to see semi-automated parts of (micro-)surgical procedures in the near future.

Conclusion

This chapter provided an overview of robotic microsurgery platforms and their clinical applications. Most available robotic systems are not particularly designed for microsurgery and therefore lack the specific requirements for this delicate type of surgery. A unique collaboration of microsurgeons and technical engineers in The Netherlands has resulted in the creation of a platform specifically designed for open microsurgery and super-microsurgery (MUSA, Microsure, The Netherlands). The evolution of this first microsurgical robot platform is described and is currently being tested in clinical studies. Robotic technology will bring microsurgery to a higher level enhancing quality and enabling new treatment possibilities. New technological developments within robotics are expected to improve microsurgical outcomes by means of precision, haptic feedback, tele-surgery, image guidance, and machine learning. Wisdom and sharing of data and technology can create great possibilities in this new era of microsurgery.

References

1. Clarke NS, Price J, Boyd T, Salizzoni S, Zehr KJ, Nieponice A, et al. Robotic-assisted microvascular surgery: skill acquisition in a rat model. J Robot Surg. 2018;12(2):331–6.
2. Dobbs TD, Cundy O, Samarendra H, Khan K, Whitaker IS. A systematic review of the role of robotics in plastic and reconstructive surgery-from inception to the future. Front Surg. 2017;4:66.
3. Tan YPA, Liverneaux P, Wong JKF. Current limitations of surgical robotics in reconstructive plastic microsurgery. Front Surg. 2018;5:22.
4. Ghanem TA. Transoral robotic-assisted microvascular reconstruction of the oropharynx. Laryngoscope. 2011;121(3):580–2.
5. Gudeloglu A, Brahmbhatt JV, Parekattil SJ. Robotic-assisted microsurgery for an elective microsurgical practice. Semin Plast Surg. 2014;28(1):11–9.
6. Ibrahim AE, Sarhane KA, Selber JC. New Frontiers in robotic-assisted microsurgical reconstruction. Clin Plast Surg. 2017;44(2):415–23.
7. Maire N, Naito K, Lequint T, Facca S, Berner S, Liverneaux P. Robot-assisted free toe pulp transfer: feasibility study. J Reconstr Microsurg. 2012;28(7):481–4.
8. Knight CG, Lorincz A, Cao A, Gidell K, Klein MD, Langenburg SE. Computer-assisted, robot-enhanced open microsurgery in an animal model. J Laparoendosc Adv Surg Tech A. 2005;15(2):182–5.
9. van der Hulst R, Sawor J, Bouvy N. Microvascular anastomosis: is there a role for robotic surgery? J Plast Reconstr Aesthet Surg. 2007;60(1):101–2.

10. van Mulken TJM, Boymans C, Schols RM, Cau R, Schoenmakers FBF, Hoekstra LT, et al. Preclinical experience using a new robotic system created for microsurgery. Plast Reconstr Surg. 2018;142(5):1367–76.
11. van Mulken TJM, Scharmga AMJ, Schols RM, Cau R, Jonis Y, Qiu SS, et al. The journey of creating the first dedicated platform for robot-assisted (super)microsurgery in reconstructive surgery. Eur J Plast Surg. 2020;43(1):1–6.
12. van Mulken TJM, Schols RM, Qiu SS, Brouwers K, Hoekstra LT, Booi DI, et al. Robotic (super) microsurgery: feasibility of a new master-slave platform in an in vivo animal model and future directions. J Surg Oncol. 2018;118(5):826–31.
13. van Mulken TJM, Schols RM, Scharmga AMJ, Winkens B, Cau R, Schoenmakers FBF, et al. First-in-human robotic supermicrosurgery using a dedicated microsurgical robot for treating breast cancer-related lymphedema: a randomized pilot trial. Nat Commun. 2020;11(1):757.
14. Cau R. Design and realization of a master-slave system for reconstructive microsurgery. Eindhoven: Technische Universiteit Eindhoven; 2014.
15. Inc TM. Titan Medical Inc. Completes Amadeus Composer(TM) Pre-Production Console and Video Tower 2013. Available from: https://titanmedicalinc.com/titan-medical-inc-completes-amadeus-composertm-pre-production-console-and-video-tower/.
16. Miroir M, Nguyen Y, Szewczyk J, Sterkers O, Bozorg Grayeli A. Design, kinematic optimization, and evaluation of a teleoperated system for middle ear microsurgery. ScientificWorldJournal. 2012;2012:907372.
17. Uneri A, Balicki MA, Handa J, Gehlbach P, Taylor RH, Iordachita I. New steady-hand eye robot with micro-force sensing for vitreoretinal surgery. Proc IEEE RAS EMBS Int Conf Biomed Robot Biomechatron. 2010;2010(26–29):814–9.
18. Maberley DAL, Beelen M, Smit J, Meenink T, Naus G, Wagner C, et al. A comparison of robotic and manual surgery for internal limiting membrane peeling. Graefes Arch Clin Exp Ophthalmol. 2020;258(4):773–8.
19. Willekens K, Gijbels A, Schoevaerdts L, Esteveny L, Janssens T, Jonckx B, et al. Robot-assisted retinal vein cannulation in an in vivo porcine retinal vein occlusion model. Acta Ophthalmol. 2017;95(3):270–5.
20. Wells TS, MacLachlan RA, Riviere CN. Toward hybrid position/force control for an active handheld micromanipulator. IEEE Int Conf Robot Autom. 2014;2014:772–7.
21. Brett P, Du X, Zoka-Assadi M, Coulson C, Reid A, Proops D. Feasibility study of a hand guided robotic drill for cochleostomy. Biomed Res Int. 2014;2014:656325.
22. Salzmann J, Zheng G, Gerber N, Stieger C, Arnold A, Rohrer U, et al. Development of a miniature robot for hearing aid implantation 2009. 2149–2154 p.
23. Dillon NP, Balachandran R, Fitzpatrick JM, Siebold MA, Labadie RF, Wanna GB, et al. A compact, bone-attached robot for Mastoidectomy. J Med Device. 2015;9(3):0310031–7.
24. Mattos L, Dagnino G, Caldwell D, Guastini L, Mora F, Peretti G. Innovations in robot-assisted laser laryngeal microsurgery 2012.
25. Feng AL, Razavi CR, Lakshminarayanan P, Ashai Z, Olds K, Balicki M, et al. The robotic ENT microsurgery system: a novel robotic platform for microvascular surgery. Laryngoscope. 2017;127(11):2495–500.
26. Sutherland GR, Wolfsberger S, Lama S, Zarei-nia K. The evolution of neuroArm. Neurosurgery. 2013;72(Suppl 1):27–32.
27. Brodie A, Vasdev N. The future of robotic surgery. Ann R Coll Surg Engl. 2018;100(Suppl 7):4–13.
28. Chen YQ, Tao JW, Su LY, Li L, Zhao SX, Yang Y, et al. Cooperative robot assistant for vitreoretinal microsurgery: development of the RVRMS and feasibility studies in an animal model. Graefes Arch Clin Exp Ophthalmol. 2017;255(6):1167–71.
29. Rahimy E, Wilson J, Tsao TC, Schwartz S, Hubschman JP. Robot-assisted intraocular surgery: development of the IRISS and feasibility studies in an animal model. Eye (Lond). 2013;27(8):972–8.

30. Gundlapalli VS, Ogunleye AA, Scott K, Wenzinger E, Ulm JP, Tavana L, et al. Robotic-assisted deep inferior epigastric artery perforator flap abdominal harvest for breast reconstruction: a case report. Microsurgery. 2018;38(6):702–5.
31. Boyd B, Umansky J, Samson M, Boyd D, Stahl K. Robotic harvest of internal mammary vessels in breast reconstruction. J Reconstr Microsurg. 2006;22(4):261–6.
32. Krapohl BD, Reichert B, Machens HG, Mailander P, Siemionow M, Zins JE. Computer-guided microsurgery: surgical evaluation of a telerobotic arm. Microsurgery. 2001;21(1):22–9.
33. Brahmbhatt JV, Gudeloglu A, Liverneaux P, Parekattil SJ. Robotic microsurgery optimization. Arch Plast Surg. 2014;41(3):225–30.
34. Narushima M, Yamamoto T, Ogata F, Yoshimatsu H, Mihara M, Koshima I. Indocyanine green Lymphography findings in limb lymphedema. J Reconstr Microsurg. 2016;32(1):72–9.
35. Loulmet D, Carpentier A, d'Attellis N, Berrebi A, Cardon C, Ponzio O, et al. Endoscopic coronary artery bypass grafting with the aid of robotic assisted instruments. J Thorac Cardiovasc Surg. 1999;118(1):4–10.
36. Reichenspurner H, Damiano RJ, Mack M, Boehm DH, Gulbins H, Detter C, et al. Use of the voice-controlled and computer-assisted surgical system ZEUS for endoscopic coronary artery bypass grafting. J Thorac Cardiovasc Surg. 1999;118(1):11–6.
37. Boyd WD, Desai ND, Kiaii B, Rayman R, Menkis AH, McKenzie FN, et al. A comparison of robot-assisted versus manually constructed endoscopic coronary anastomosis. Ann Thorac Surg. 2000;70(3):839–42. discussion 42–3
38. Boyd WD, Rayman R, Desai ND, Menkis AH, Dobkowski W, Ganapathy S, et al. Closed-chest coronary artery bypass grafting on the beating heart with the use of a computer-enhanced surgical robotic system. J Thorac Cardiovasc Surg. 2000;120(4):807–9.
39. O'Malley BW Jr, Weinstein GS, Hockstein NG. Transoral robotic surgery (TORS): glottic microsurgery in a canine model. J Voice. 2006;20(2):263–8.
40. Hockstein NG, Nolan JP, O'Malley BW Jr, Woo YJ. Robot-assisted pharyngeal and laryngeal microsurgery: results of robotic cadaver dissections. Laryngoscope. 2005;115(6):1003–8.
41. Kazmitcheff G, Nguyen Y, Miroir M, Pean F, Ferrary E, Cotin S, et al. Middle-ear microsurgery simulation to improve new robotic procedures. Biomed Res Int. 2014;2014:891742.
42. Chammas J, Sauer A, Pizzuto J, Pouthier F, Gaucher D, Marescaux J, et al. Da Vinci Xi robot-assisted penetrating Keratoplasty. Transl Vis Sci Technol. 2017;6(3):21.
43. Bourcier T, Becmeur PH, Mutter D. Robotically assisted amniotic membrane transplant surgery. JAMA Ophthalmol. 2015;133(2):213–4.
44. Edwards TL, Xue K, Meenink HCM, Beelen MJ, Naus GJL, Simunovic MP, et al. First-in-human study of the safety and viability of intraocular robotic surgery. Nat Biomed Eng. 2018;2:649–56.
45. Latif MJ, Afthinos JN, Connery CP, Perin N, Bhora FY, Chwajol M, et al. Robotic intercostal nerve graft for reversal of thoracic sympathectomy: a large animal feasibility model. Int J Med Robot. 2008;4(3):258–62.
46. Gözen A, Tokas T, Tawfick A, Mousa WEM, Kotb M, Tzanaki E, et al. Robot-assisted vaso-vasostomy and vasoepididymostomy: current status and review of the literature. Turk J Urol. 2020;46(5):329–34.
47. Dickey RM, Pastuszak AW, Hakky TS, Chandrashekar A, Ramasamy R, Lipshultz LI. The evolution of vasectomy reversal. Curr Urol Rep. 2015;16(6):40.
48. Parekattil SJ, Gudeloglu A. Robotic assisted andrological surgery. Asian J Androl. 2013;15(1):67–74.
49. Katz RD, Rosson GD, Taylor JA, Singh NK. Robotics in microsurgery: use of a surgical robot to perform a free flap in a pig. Microsurgery. 2005;25(7):566–9.
50. Selber JC. Transoral robotic reconstruction of oropharyngeal defects: a case series. Plast Reconstr Surg. 2010;126(6):1978–87.
51. Selber JC, Baumann DP, Holsinger FC. Robotic latissimus dorsi muscle harvest: a case series. Plast Reconstr Surg. 2012;129(6):1305–12.
52. Selber JC. The robotic DIEP flap. Plast Reconstr Surg. 2020;145(2):340–3.

53. Struk S, Sarfati B, Leymarie N, Missistrano A, Alkhashnam H, Rimareix F, et al. Robotic-assisted DIEP flap harvest: a feasibility study on cadaveric model. J Plast Reconstr Aesthet Surg. 2018;71(2):259–61.
54. Masia J, Olivares L, Koshima I, Teo TC, Suominen S, Van Landuyt K, et al. Barcelona consensus on supermicrosurgery. J Reconstr Microsurg. 2014;30(1):53–8.
55. Koshima I, Inagawa K, Urushibara K, Moriguchi T. Supermicrosurgical lymphaticovenular anastomosis for the treatment of lymphedema in the upper extremities. J Reconstr Microsurg. 2000;16(6):437–42.
56. Zhang D, Chen J, Li W, Bautista Salinas D, Yang GZ. A microsurgical robot research platform for robot-assisted microsurgery research and training. Int J Comput Assist Radiol Surg. 2020;15(1):15–25.
57. Schols RM, Connell NJ, Stassen LP. Near-infrared fluorescence imaging for real-time intraoperative anatomical guidance in minimally invasive surgery: a systematic review of the literature. World J Surg. 2015;39(5):1069–79.
58. Lee BT, Matsui A, Hutteman M, Lin SJ, Winer JH, Laurence RG, et al. Intraoperative near-infrared fluorescence imaging in perforator flap reconstruction: current research and early clinical experience. J Reconstr Microsurg. 2010;26(1):59–65.

Index

Printed in the United States
by Baker & Taylor Publisher Services